KU-505-751

Medical Genetics for the MRCOG and Beyond

J Michael Connor DSc MD FRCP
Professor of Medical Genetics, University of Glasgow,
Division of Developmental Medicine, Institute of Medical
Genetics, Yorkhill Hospitals, Glasgow G3 8SJ, UK

RCOG Press

Published by the **RCOG Press**
at the Royal College of Obstetricians and Gynaecologists,
27 Sussex Place, Regent's Park, London NW1 4RG

www.rcog.org.uk

Registered charity no. 213280

First published 2005

© The Royal College of Obstetricians and Gynaecologists

No part of this publication may be reproduced, stored or transmitted in any form or by any means, without the prior written permission of the publisher or, in the case of reprographic reproduction, in accordance with the terms of licences issued by the Copyright Licensing Agency in the UK [www.cla.co.uk]. Enquiries concerning reproduction outside the terms stated here should be sent to the publisher at the UK address printed on this page.

The use of registered names, trademarks, etc. in this publication does not imply, even in the absence of a specific statement, that such names are exempt from the relevant laws and regulations and therefore for general use.

While every effort has been made to ensure the accuracy of the information contained within this publication, the publisher can give no guarantee for information about drug dosage and application thereof contained in this book. In every individual case the respective user must check current indications and accuracy by consulting other pharmaceutical literature and following the guidelines laid down by the manufacturers of specific products and the relevant authorities in the country in which they are practising.

The publisher can give no guarantee for information about drug dosage and application thereof contained in this book. In every individual case the respective user must check its accuracy by consulting other pharmaceutical literature.

The right of Michael Connor to be identified as Author of this work has been asserted by him in accordance with the Copyright, Designs and Patents Act, 1988.

ISBN 1 900364 99 9

Cover illustration: Genes of female with translocation between chromosomes 13 and 18

RCOG Editor: Jane Moody
Design/typesetting by Karl Harrington, FiSH Books
Printed by Latimer Trend & Co. Ltd., Estover Road, Plymouth PL6 7PL, UK

Contents

Abbreviations   vii

Glossary   ix

Preface   xv

**Section One: General principles of medical
genetics**   1
Introduction   3
Normal human inheritance   3
Types of genetic disease   5
Drawing the family tree   19
Interpreting the family tree   22
DNA analysis   24
Chromosome analysis   28
Referral for genetic assessment and counselling   30

**Section Two: Common genetic problems in
obstetric and gynaecological practice**   33
Introduction   35
Genetic causes of infertility   35
Genetic causes of recurrent miscarriages   36
Elevated maternal screening risk   41
Family history   52

Section Three: Clinical case scenarios   67
Introduction   69
Case 1:   Unexpected finding at amniocentesis   69
Case 2:   Lethal short-limbed skeletal dysplasia   71
Case 3:   Family history of Down syndrome   71
Case 4:   Family history of Huntington's disease   72
Case 5:   Family history of Duchenne muscular
          dystrophy   73
Case 6:   Unexplained high level of maternal serum
          alphafetoprotein   74
Case 7:   Family history of siblings with Goldenhar
          syndrome   74
Case 8:   Family history of microcephaly   75

Case 9: Unexpected finding at amniocentesis 76
Case 10: Family history of Down syndrome 77
Case 11: Importance of genetic ancestry 77
Case 12: Never say never 79
Case 13: Unexpected finding at amniocentesis 80
Case 14: Inherited limb abnormality 81
Case 15: Multiple congenital abnormalities 83
Case 16: Family history of cystic fibrosis 84
Case 17: Previous obstetric history of trisomy 13 85
Case 18: Previous obstetric history of hydrocephalus 86
Case 19: Maternal congenital heart disease 89
Case 20: Family history of problems 89
Case 21: Unexpected findings at amniocentesis 91
Case 22: Previous obstetric history of a fetus with
multiple congenital malformations 92
Case 23: Accidental X-ray in early pregnancy 93
Case 24: Genetic mimicry 94
Case 25: Previous obstetric history on an intrauterine
death with cystic hygroma 95

Appendix 1: Sources of genetic information 97

Further reading 99

Index 100

Abbreviations

A	adenine
α-FP	alphafetoprotein
bp	base pair
BRCA1	breast cancer type 1 gene
C	cytosine
CFTR	cystic fibrosis transmembrane conductance regulator gene
CPK	creatine phosphokinase
CVS	chorionic villus sampling
DMD	Duchenne muscular dystrophy
DMPK	dystrophia myotonica protein kinase gene
DNA	deoxyribonucleic acid
EDTA	ethylenediamine tetra-acetic acid
FβhCG	free beta human chorionic gonadotrophin
FMR1	fragile site mental retardation 1 gene
G	guanine
Gy	gray
hCG	human chorionic gonadotrophin
HPRT	hypoxanthine phosphoribosyltransferase gene
IDUA	alpha-L-iduronidase gene
kb	kilobase
L1CAM	L1 cell adhesion molecule gene
Mb	megabase
M/M	mutant/mutant

MOM	multiples of the median
MSα-FP	maternal serum alphafetoprotein
N/M	normal/mutant
PAPP-A	pregnancy-associated plasma protein A
PCR	polymerase chain reaction
rads	radiation absorbed doses
T	thymine
TP73L	tumour protein p73-like gene

Glossary

allele	alternative forms of a gene at the same locus
autosomal dominant inheritance	mutation in one member of an autosomal gene pair results in disease
autosomal recessive inheritance	mutation in both members of an autosomal gene pair is necessary for disease to occur
autosome	chromosomes numbers 1 to 22 inclusive
balanced translocation	transfer of chromosomal material between chromosomes with no overall gain or loss and hence no clinical effect
base pair	unit of length of DNA of one set of paired bases (AT or GC)
carrier	a person with one mutation in an autosomal gene pair which shows autosomal recessive inheritance (i.e. no clinical effect unless both members of the gene pair are mutated)
centromere	a constricted area of the chromosome which divides it into short and long arms
chromosome disorder	any abnormality of chromosome number or structure visible under the light microscope
codon	three consecutive bases in DNA (or RNA) which specify an amino acid
congenital	present at birth
consanguineous	mating between individuals who share at least one common ancestor
consultand	a person requesting genetic counselling

deletion	loss of chromosomal material
diagnostic test	a test which confirms or refutes a diagnosis
dizygotic twins	twins which arise from the fertilisation of two separate eggs
dominant	a trait expressed in the heterozygote
empiric risk	recurrence risk based on experience rather than calculation
false negative rate	proportion of affected cases missed by a screening test
first-degree relatives	immediate relatives who have one half of their genes in common (e.g. parent and child or brother and sister)
gene	a segment of DNA which codes for a functional product (e.g. a protein)
gene probe	a labelled segment of DNA which can be used to find its matching segment amongst a mixture of DNA fragments
genetic counselling	communication of information and advice about inherited disorders
genetic heterogeneity	genetic mimicry where mutations in different genes can produce a similar clinical picture
genomic imprinting	parent-specific expression or repression of genes in offspring
genotype	the genetic make-up of an individual
gonadal mosaic	a person with a mixture of cells in their gonad, some with a mutation and some without
heterozygous	a person with a gene pair which has one mutant and one normal gene
homozygous	a person with a gene pair in which both copies of the gene are mutant or normal
independent risks	risks where the outcome of one event has no influence on the outcome of the other

	(e.g. if two coins are tossed heads or tails may occur for either and the result for one does not influence the other)
karyotype	the chromosomal make-up of an individual
kilobase	a unit of length of DNA of 1000 base pairs
length mutation	a type of DNA change where the DNA sequence is increased or decreased in size
locus	the location of a gene on a chromosome
megabase	a unit of length of DNA of 1 000 000 base pairs
meiosis	reduction cell division which occurs in the gonads in the production of eggs and sperm
microdeletion	a chromosomal deletion which is at or below the limit of resolution using a light microscope
mitosis	normal cell division which results in daughter cells with an identical genetic complement
monozygotic twins	twins which result from the early division of a single fertilised egg into two embryos
mosaic	an individual with cells with two or more genetic constitutions
multifactorial inheritance	conditions arising from the interaction of multiple genes and environmental factors
mutation	alteration of genetic material
mutational heterogeneity	different mutations in a particular gene may cause the same disease
mutually exclusive risks	risks where one outcome of an event precludes another outcome (e.g. a single tossed coin can result in heads or tails but not both)

non-penetrance	no signs or symptoms in an individual who has inherited an autosomal dominant trait
point mutation	a type of DNA change where a single base is replaced with another base
phenotype	the clinical features of an individual
polymerase chain reaction	a technique for amplification of a target segment of DNA
polymorphism	a common DNA or chromosomal variant (present in at least 2% of the population)
proband	the individual who draws medical attention to the family
recessive	a trait which is expressed only in homozygotes
satellite stalks	the short arms of chromosomes 13,14, 15, 21 and 22
screening test	a test which divides a population according to risk for a condition; those at high risk are then offered a diagnostic test
second-degree relatives	close relatives with one-quarter of their genes in common (e.g. grandparent and grandchild or nephew/niece and aunt/uncle)
sensitivity	the proportion of cases detected by a screening test
sibship	a family group of brothers and/or sisters
somatic cell genetic disorders	conditions which arise after conception from a cumulation of genetic mutations in a cell or group of cells
somatic mosaic	a person with a mixture of cells, some with a mutation and some without
specificity	the proportion of the unaffected population included by a screening test in the high-risk group (also called the false positive rate)

syndrome	a non-random combination of clinical features
telomere	the ends of the short and long arms of the chromosomes
third-degree relatives	more distant relatives who share one-eighth of their genes (e.g. first cousins)
trait	any gene-determined characteristic
translocation	the transfer of chromosomal material between chromosomes
triploidy	an extra half set of chromosomes resulting in 69 in total
trisomy	an extra copy of a chromosome resulting in 47 in total
variable expression	variation in clinical effects of an autosomal dominant trait
X-linked recessive inheritance	disease due to mutations in genes on the X-chromosome; males with only one X are affected if that copy is mutant whereas females with two X chromosomes are usually unaffected if only one copy is mutant

Preface

There is a long history of successful interaction between obstetrics and gynaecology and medical genetics. Initially, most applications related to obstetrics, especially with the use of prenatal diagnosis and prenatal screening but, more recently, the growth has been in applications related to gynaecology, especially in relation to gynaecological malignancies.

However, despite this long history, there is a widespread misconception that genetics is a difficult subject to understand. This book thus aims to dispel this misconception as well as providing a revision aid for the MRCOG candidate. The first section covers basic principles. The second section outlines the more common situations where obstetrics and gynaecology and medical genetics interact and the third section contains real-life clinical case scenarios. These scenarios have been selected to represent typical problems and to highlight areas which, if mismanaged, could (and did, in these cases) lead to medico-legal consequences.

Michael Connor
December 2004

Section One

General principles of medical genetics

General principles of medical genetics

Introduction

This section summarises the basic principles of normal inheritance and genetic disease and outlines the approaches for identification of people with or without risk factors for a genetic disorder.

Normal human inheritance

Medical genetics is concerned with human biological variation as it relates to health and disease. This variation may be due to inherited genetic information (nature) or due to environmental factors (nurture). It can also result from combinations of these two influences. The genetic information is coded in DNA, which is packaged into chromosomes. Each chromosome contains a single DNA molecule consisting of two strands woven together as a double helix. Each nucleus has 46 chromosomes; these can be arranged into a karyotype of matching pairs, starting with the largest (numbered 1) down to the smallest (numbered 22) (Figure 1.1). This leaves the sex chromosomes, which are two X chromosomes in a female (Figure 1.1) and an X and a Y in a male (Figure 1.2). When an individual reproduces, only one of each pair will be transmitted to the egg or the sperm. Thus, each egg has only 23 chromosomes (1–22 and an X). Each sperm similarly has 23 chromosomes with one of each pair, 1–22 and either the X or the Y chromosome. Fusion of the egg and sperm restores the full complement of 46 chromosomes and establishes the sex of the embryo.

DNA is composed of four types of bases: adenine (A), cytosine (C), guanine (G) and thymine (T). These bases show specific pairing between the DNA strands of the double helix. A pairs with T and G pairs with C. The unit of length of DNA is a base pair (bp) of AT or CG. One thousand base pairs is a kilobase (kb) and one million base pairs is a megabase (Mb). The chromosomes vary in size and contain different amounts of DNA, from 280 Mb in each copy of chromosome 1, to 45 Mb in each copy of chromosome 21.

Information is stored in DNA using the sequence of bases (A, T, C or G) along a DNA strand. These bases are read three at a time as a

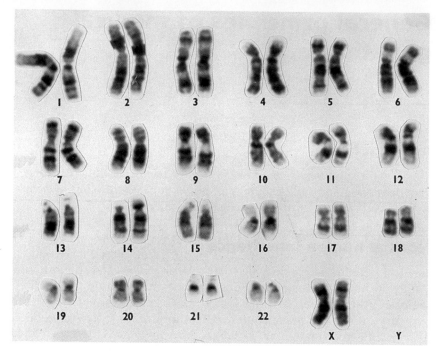

Figure 1.1 Normal female karyotype

codon and this provides 64 (4^3) combinations. This is more than enough to code for the 20 amino acids which are used to make all proteins and to code for stop and start signals for protein synthesis. The region of the DNA that codes for a particular protein is defined as its gene. Genes vary greatly in size; small genes may be under 1 kb in size, while enormous genes may be over one megabase in size. Some areas of the DNA between genes may have roles in regulation of gene function but large areas of human DNA (perhaps as much as 30% of the total) have no known function.

In total, 30 000 genes are encoded in human DNA. Most of these have now been identified and their DNA sequence determined, at least in part. Some genes are unique (with a single copy in each chromosome) whereas others are repeated, with multiple copies that may be adjacent or scattered. The genes are not evenly distributed throughout the chromosomes. The dark banded areas of the chromosomes in Figures 1.1 and 1.2 are relatively 'gene poor' compared with the lighter banded areas. More genes are found towards the ends of the chromosomes (telomeres) than around the central constrictions (centromeres).

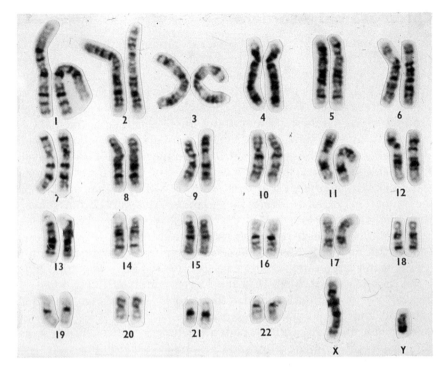

Figure 1.2 Normal male karyotype

Types of genetic disease

With the exception of identical twins, individuals vary. This variation reflects inherited genetic factors, environmental influences and their interaction. In medical genetics, there are often difficulties in defining the boundary between 'normal' genetic variation and 'mild' genetic disease. It can also be hard to disentangle the influences of one gene on another and of environmental factors on genes. The subdivision into various types of genetic disease is therefore somewhat artificial and the frequency of each group of genetic diseases depends upon where the boundaries between normality and disease are placed. Traditionally, genetic diseases are subdivided into:

- chromosomal disorders
- single gene disorders
- multifactorial disorders
- somatic cell genetic disorders.

Chromosomal disorders

By definition, a chromosomal disorder is present if there is a visible alteration in the number or structure of the chromosomes. These changes may affect either the sex chromosomes (X or Y) or the autosomes (numbers 1–22). Using routine light microscopy, multiple newborn cytogenetic surveys have revealed a frequency of six chromosomal disorders per 1000 births. Of these six, two-thirds are disabled, either mentally or physically, as a result. These liveborn infants with chromosomal abnormalities comprise only a small proportion of all chromosomally abnormal conceptions. It is estimated that the rate of chromosomal abnormality in embryonic and fetal deaths is within the range 32–42%; the proportion of all recognised conceptuses that are chromosomally abnormal is thus 5–7%.

Normally, each sperm and egg has 23 chromosomes, with one of each pair of autosomes (1–22) and one sex chromosome. Malsegregation is common and can result in an egg or a sperm with either an extra copy of a chromosome (24 in total) or a missing chromosome (22 in total). In general, loss of chromosomal material is more serious than additional material and autosomal imbalances are more serious than sex chromosome imbalances. In consequence, different types of chromosomal abnormality predominate in miscarriages and in liveborn infants.

Additional copies of any autosome in the egg or sperm will result in 47 chromosomes in the fetus and these will generally result in miscarriage. For example, an extra copy of chromosome 16 (trisomy 16) is the most common autosomal trisomy in miscarriages, whereas trisomies for chromosome 21 (Down syndrome, Figure 1.3), 18 (Edwards syndrome, Figure 1.4) and 13 (Patau syndrome, Figure 1.5) are the most common trisomies in liveborn infants.

A missing autosome usually results in a very early pregnancy failure and is undetected. However, monosomy X with a single copy of the X and 45 chromosomes in total (45,X, Figure 1.6) occurs in approximately 1% of all conceptions; 98% of these pregnancies are spontaneously miscarried. This high *in utero* lethality contrasts with the relatively mild postnatal features of children with 45,X (Turner syndrome).

An extra half set of chromosomes results from fertilisation of an egg by two sperm and leads to 69 chromosomes in total (triploidy, Figure 1.7). Triploidy usually results in a miscarriage but, exceptionally, infants may be liveborn.

Structural aberrations result from chromosomal breakage. When a chromosome breaks, two unstable sticky ends are produced. Generally, repair mechanisms rejoin these two ends. However, if more than one break has occurred then, as the repair mechanisms cannot distinguish one

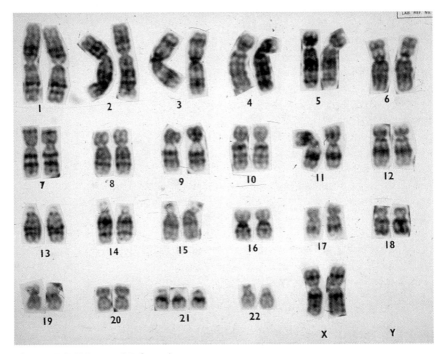

Figure 1.3 Trisomy 21 female

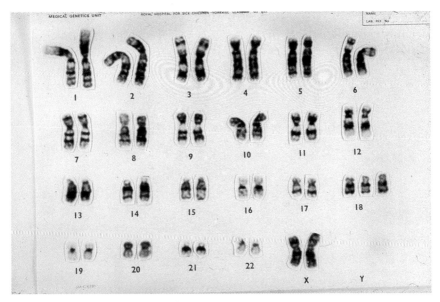

Figure 1.4 Trisomy 18 female

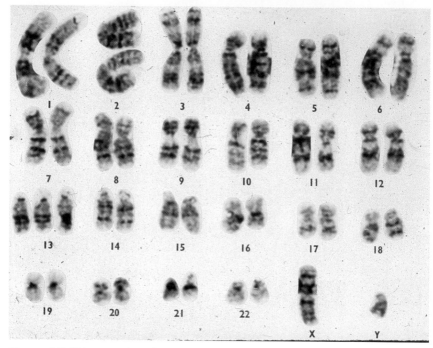

Figure 1.5 Trisomy 13 male

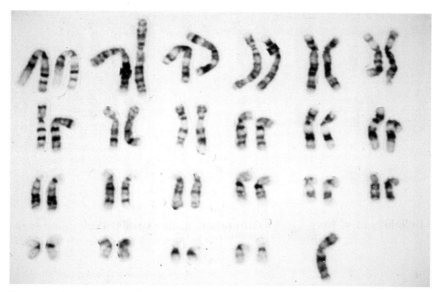

Figure 1.6 Turner syndrome: 45,X

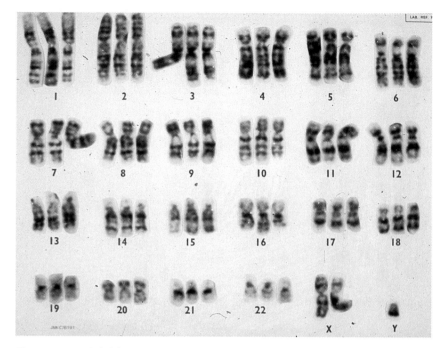

Figure 1.7 Triploidy: 69,XXY

sticky end from another, there is the possibility of joining the wrong ends. The most common types of structural aberrations are translocations and deletions.

Translocations involve the transfer of chromosomal material between chromosomes. The process requires simultaneous breakage of two chromosomes, which then repair in an abnormal arrangement (Figure 1.8). This exchange can involve any two chromosomes and usually results in no loss of vital DNA. In this case, the individual is clinically normal and is said to have a balanced translocation. The medical significance is its relevance for future generations, because a balanced translocation carrier is at risk of producing chromosomally unbalanced offspring. The overall frequency of translocations in the general population is 2:1000.

Deletions arise from loss of chromosomal material between two break points on the same chromosome. They can also result from a parent with a balanced translocation. Visible deletions of the autosomes always produce clinical effects, which commonly include learning disabilities, congenital malformations and unusual facial features. Submicroscopic deletions are also clinically important. The smallest visible change to a

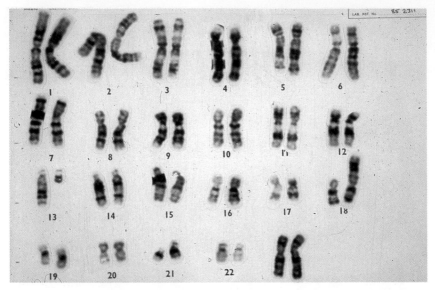

Figure 1.8 Female with a translocation between chromosomes 13 and 18

chromosome using the light microscope approximates to the loss of 4 Mb of DNA. Smaller losses can easily include multiple genes and a large number of microdeletion syndromes have now been identified using DNA probes for the deleted area (Table 1.1).

Single-gene disorders

Single-gene disorders (Mendelian disorders) are due to mutations in one or both members of a pair of autosomal genes or to mutations in single genes on the X or Y chromosomes. Within each chromosome the genes have a strict order, with each gene occupying a specific location or locus. Thus, the autosomal genes are present in pairs, one on the maternally inherited copy of the pair and the other on the paternal copy. Alternative forms of a gene are called alleles and these arise by mutation of the normal allele and may or may not have an altered function. If both members of a gene pair are identical then the individual is said to be homozygous (noun – homozygote) for that locus and if different the individual is said to be heterozygous (noun – heterozygote).

Any gene-determined characteristic is called a trait. If a trait is expressed in the heterozygote then the trait is described as dominant, whereas if it is only expressed in the homozygote then it is described as recessive.

Table 1.1 Examples of chromosomal microdeletion syndromes

Disorder	Region of microdeletion[a]
Alagille syndrome	20p
Angelman syndrome	15q11-12
DiGeorge syndrome	22q11
Miller-Dieker lissencephaly	17p13
Prader–Willi syndrome	15q11-12
Williams syndrome	7q
Wilms tumour, aniridia syndrome	11p13

[a] p represents the short arm of a chromosome, which is above the centromere in the karyotype; q represents the long arm of a chromosome, which is below the centromere in the karyotype

Hence, all single-gene disorders may be classified according to their chromosomal location (autosomal, X-linked or Y-linked) and further subdivided into dominant and recessive (Table 1.2).

Table 1.2 Examples of single-gene disorders (in approximate frequency order)

Trait	Single-gene disorders
Autosomal dominant	Inherited colon cancer, inherited breast cancer, dominant otosclerosis, familial hypercholesterolaemia, von Willebrand's disease, adult polycystic kidney disease, neurofibromatosis, myotonic dystrophy, Huntington's disease, tuberous sclerosis
Autosomal recessive	Cystic fibrosis, recessive learning disabilities (multiple subtypes), congenital deafness (multiple subtypes), phenylketonuria, spinal muscular atrophy
X-linked dominant	Xg blood group, vitamin D-resistant rickets, hereditary motor and sensory neuropathy (one type), incontinentia pigmenti, Rett syndrome
X-linked recessive	Red-green colour blindness, fragile X syndrome, non-specific X-linked learning disabilities (several subtypes), Duchenne muscular dystrophy, haemophilia A, X-linked ichthyosis
Y-linked	Male sex determination

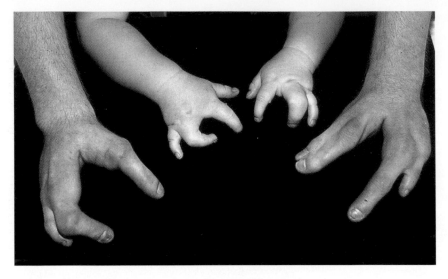

Figure 1.9 Father and daughter with split-hand syndrome (ectrodactyly)

AUTOSOMAL DOMINANT INHERITANCE

Autosomal dominant inheritance is illustrated by the condition shown in Figure 1.9. In this family, the father and daughter have deformed hands and feet with longitudinal splitting, which is called ectrodactyly. This condition is inherited as an autosomal dominant trait and, in this family, it is caused by a mutation in one copy of the paired autosomal genes called *TP73L* (tumour protein p73-like). This gene is located on the long arm of chromosome 3. Each affected person has a single underactive copy and is affected despite the normal copy of this gene on the opposite copy of chromosome 3, which was inherited from the other parent. The risk of an affected person transmitting the copy of chromosome 3 with the mutated gene is one in two (Figure 1.10).

AUTOSOMAL RECESSIVE INHERITANCE

Autosomal recessive inheritance is illustrated by the condition shown in Figure 1.11. In this family, the parents and other relatives are healthy but one of their children has learning disabilities due to Hurler syndrome. Hurler syndrome is inherited as an autosomal recessive trait and is caused by a mutation in both copies of the alpha-L-iduronidase gene (symbolised *IDUA*) located on the tip of the short arm of chromosome 4. The affected child has two copies of the mutant gene whereas

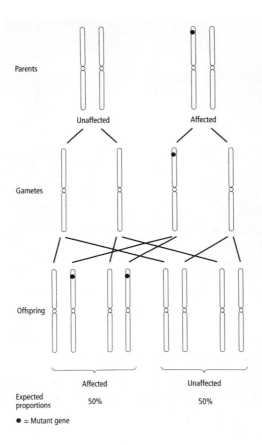

Parents

Unaffected   Affected

Gametes

Offspring

Affected   Unaffected

Expected
proportions   50%   50%

● = Mutant gene

Figure 1.10 Diagram of autosomal dominant inheritance

the normal parents have a single mutant copy and a normal gene on the opposite copy of chromosome 4 and are termed carriers or hetero-zygotes. For two carrier parents the chance of further affected children is on average one in four (Figure 1.12).

X-LINKED RECESSIVE INHERITANCE

X-linked recessive inheritance is illustrated by the condition shown in Figure 1.13. The boy shown in the figure has learning disabilities caused by Lesch–Nyhan syndrome. This is caused by a mutation in the *HPRT* gene on the long arm of the X chromosome. Males with a single mutant *HPRT* gene are affected, as the partner sex chromosome (Y) does not

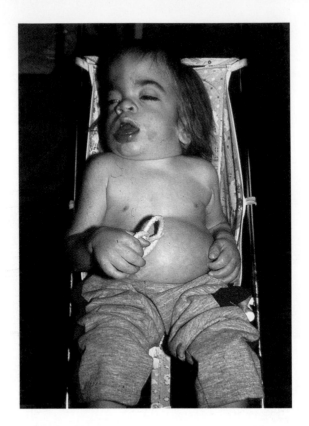

Figure 1.11 Hurler syndrome

have a copy of this gene. Females with a single mutant *HPRT* gene are healthy owing to the presence of the normal *HPRT* gene on their other X chromosome. Such a female, with one normal and one mutant copy, is termed a carrier and she has a one in two chance of transmitting the X chromosome incorporating the mutant gene to the next generation. The sex of each child is determined by the sex chromosome transmitted by the father. There is a one in two chance that the Y chromosome will be transmitted resulting in a male and a one in two chance that the X chromosome will be transmitted resulting in a female. Thus, for a carrier mother half of her sons will be affected and half of her daughters will be carriers (Figure 1.14).

The overall frequency of single-gene diseases is not known. An early estimate, which is now known to be much too low, gave a combined frequency of 10:1000 (7:1000 autosomal dominant, 2.5:1000 autosomal recessive, 0.5:1000 X-linked recessive). The number of recognised single-

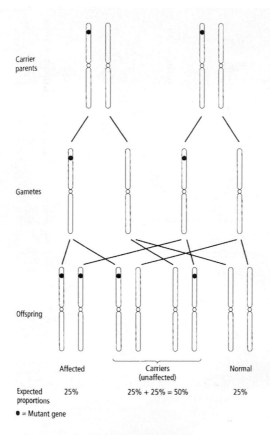

Figure 1.12 Diagram of autosomal recessive inheritance

gene traits has since more than quadrupled to over 12 000 and includes several common conditions such as familial breast cancer and familial colon cancer, which each affect 5:1000). In addition, DNA analysis has revealed higher than expected frequencies of generally asymptomatic people with one or two mutant alleles at a locus. For example, up to 1% of the population has a mutant allele for von Willebrand coagulation factor and yet most are asymptomatic.

Multifactorial (or part-genetic) disorders

Multifactorial disorders result from an interaction of one or more genes with one or more environmental factors. In effect, the genetic contribution predisposes the individual to the actions of environmental agents.

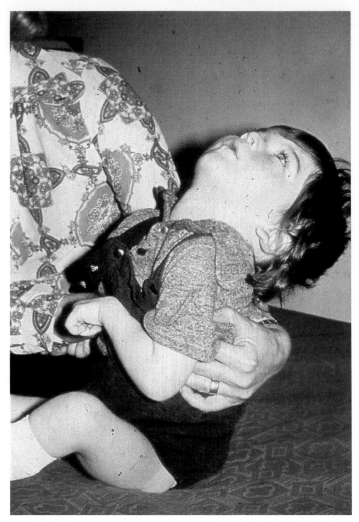

Figure 1.13 Lesch–Nyhan syndrome

Such an interaction is suspected when conditions show an increased recurrence risk within families, which does not reach the level of risk seen for single-gene disorders. In contrast to single-gene disorders, the pedigree pattern is not diagnostic for multifactorial disorders and proof of this pattern of inheritance usually rests on twin studies.

Identical (or monozygotic) twins have 100% of their genes in common whereas non-identical (dizygotic) twins have only 50% of their genes in common. If a condition has no genetic influence then the frequencies in

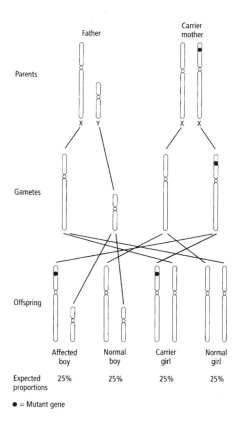

Parents

Father

Carrier mother

X Y

X X

Gametes

Offspring

| Affected boy | Normal boy | Carrier girl | Normal girl |

Expected proportions 25% 25% 25% 25%

● = Mutant gene

Figure 1.14 Diagram of X-linked recessive inheritance

identical and non-identical twins should be comparable. For multifactorial disorders, the frequency in identical twins is higher than in non-identical twins but is not as high as the 100% figure seen with single-gene disorders. Thus, for example, the likelihood that both non-identical twins will be affected with multifactorial cleft lip and palate is 5%, whereas for identical twins the comparable figure is 35%.

Multifactorial disorders are believed to account for approximately 50% of all congenital malformations and are thought to be relevant to many common chronic disorders of adulthood, including hypertension, rheumatoid arthritis, schizophrenia, manic depression, multiple sclerosis, diabetes mellitus, premature vascular disease and senile dementia. The collective frequency of multifactorial malformations is estimated at 45:1000 live births and the collective frequency of multifactorial common disorders of adulthood may be as high as 600:1000 over a lifetime. In addition, multifactorial inheritance is suspected for many common psychological disorders of childhood, including dyslexia, specific language impairment and attention deficit hyperactivity disorder. Hence, multifactorial disease represents the most common type of genetic disease in both children and adults.

Somatic cell (or cumulative) genetic disorders

When a mutation is present in the fertilised egg it will be transmitted to all daughter cells, including the germ cells. If, however, a mutation arises after the first cell division, this mutation will only be found in a proportion of cells and the individual is said to be mosaic. The mutation may be confined to the gonadal cells (gonadal mosaic) or to the somatic cells (somatic mosaic) or may occur in a proportion of both.

Cancers are somatic cell genetic disorders. The initiating event for each cancer is the occurrence of one or more key mutations in the same somatic cell. With progression, further genetic changes accumulate in the cancerous cells and can include mutations in other genes as well as numerical and structural chromosomal abnormalities (Figure 1.15). These changes are confined to the somatic cells of the tumour and not the gonadal cells, so the condition is not inherited and the risks to family members are not increased above the general population risk.

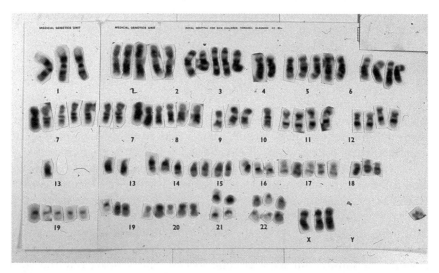

Figure 1.15 Multiple numerical and structural chromosomal aberrations in a rhabdomyosarcoma

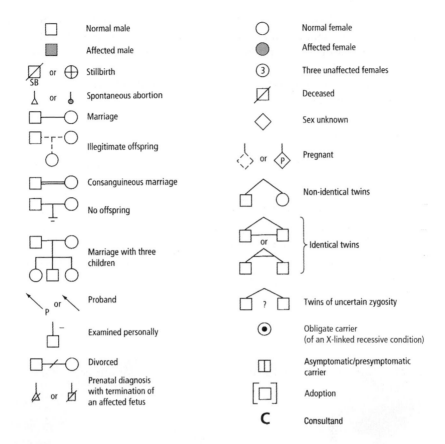

Figure 1.16 Symbols used for pedigree construction

For some rare cancers and in some families with common cancers, the first step in the cascade of mutations may be inherited. In this situation, the condition is inherited as a single-gene disorder, with high risks to other family members.

Non-inherited cancers are common, with a lifetime risk of 250:1000. Somatic cell genetic disorders might also be involved in other clinical conditions such as autoimmune disorders and the aging process.

Drawing the family tree

Normally, a family will see a genetic specialist after being referred by a general practitioner, another specialist or a member of one of the professions allied to medicine. The referring healthcare professional may have the genetic basis of a condition brought to his or her attention by a patient or may find a clinical sign suggestive of a genetic disorder on examination. Once alerted to the possibility of a genetic disorder, even the non-geneticist should draw a family tree. This is done freehand, using a standard set of symbols (Figure 1.16).

The family tree, or pedigree, is a compact way of storing a large amount of family information. Each generation occupies the same horizontal level and within a generation the birth order is presented from left to right. It is usually easiest to start with the youngest generation at the bottom of the page and then work back to older generations. For each member of the pedigree, name and age are usually included. Miscarriages, neonatal deaths, children with physical or learning disabilities and parental consanguinity might not be mentioned unless specifically asked about.

The newborn child shown in Figure 1.17 has bilateral polydactyly. The family history taken at admission for delivery is shown in Figure 1.18. The family tree was then taken properly and this revealed multiple affected individuals in several generations, including the child's mother (Figures 1.19 and 1.20).

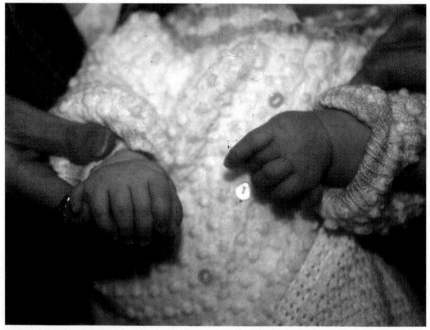

Figure 1.17 Bilateral postaxial (little finger side) polydactyly

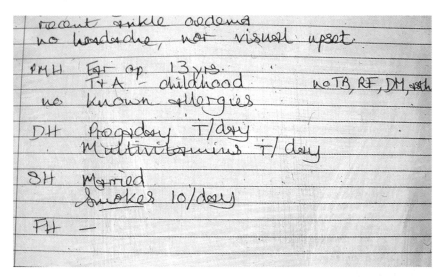

recent ankle oedema
no headache, nor visual upset.

PMH Ear op 13yrs.
     T+A - childhood   noTB, RF, DM, asth
no known allergies

DH Progesdasy T/day
    Multivitamins T/day

SH Married
    Smokes 10/day

FH —

Figure 1.18 How not to take a family history

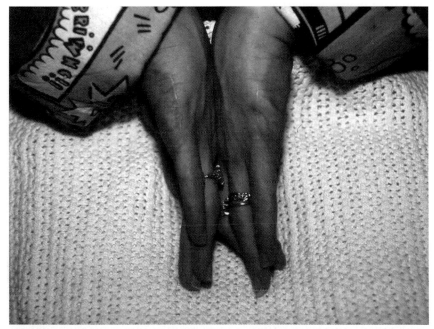

Figure 1.19 Mother of the child in Figure 1.17, with scars where her extra digits were removed

Interpreting the family tree

In the family with polydactyly shown in Figure 1.20, both males and females are affected and so the gene causing polydactyly cannot be on the Y chromosome. There is also an instance of a male passing it on to a male. Since a male does not transmit an X chromosome to his sons, we can conclude that the polydactyly gene is not on the X chromosome and therefore it must be on one of the autosomes.

Looking at the family, it would be extremely unlikely that the partners of affected people were, by chance, carriers of the polydactyly gene and so affected children must have received only a single copy of the abnormal gene from the affected parent. Since they have developed polydactyly even though they have inherited a healthy gene from the other parent, the polydactyly copy of the gene is said to be dominant to the healthy copy of the gene. Polydactyly in this family is thus inherited as an autosomal dominant trait.

Each affected person with this or any other autosomal dominant trait is thus heterozygous, with one normal and one mutant gene at this genetic location. The affected person will pass on either the normal or the mutant gene and so the risk to each child is one in two (Figure 1.10).

In a family tree, the following features help to confirm the autosomal dominant mode of inheritance:

- There are usually affected people in each generation with passage from one affected person to another (this is termed a vertical pattern of inheritance).

- Men and women are equally likely to be affected and, if affected, have a similar severity.

- Men can transmit the condition to sons or daughters.

- Women can transmit the condition to sons or daughters.

- On average one-half of the children of an affected person will be affected.

Figure 1.21 shows a different pattern of inheritance. In contrast to the previous example, affected people are present in only one sibship, that is, a family group of brothers and sisters, in one generation. This is called a horizontal pattern of inheritance. The parents are unaffected but may be blood relatives (consanguineous). Men and women may be affected but with a low risk to their own offspring.

Another pattern of inheritance can be seen in Figure 1.22. In contrast to the autosomal dominant and autosomal recessive patterns, only males are affected. Affected men occur in more than one generation and are linked to each other by healthy women (this is termed a knight's move

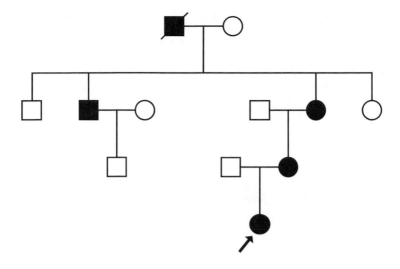

Figure 1.20 Pedigree of mother and child in Figures 1.17 and 1.19

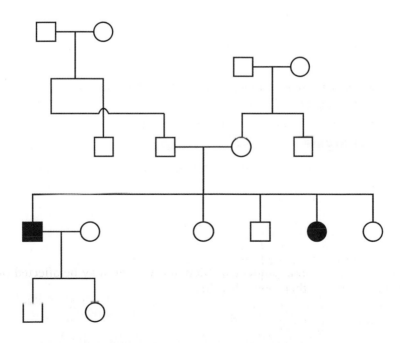

Figure 1.21 Example of an autosomal recessive family tree

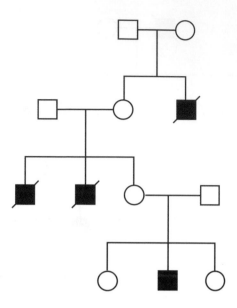

Figure 1.22 Example of an X-linked recessive family tree

pattern of inheritance). Affected men never transmit the trait to their sons (that is, there is no male-to-male transmission). The women who link affected males are termed obligate carriers, as they must be heterozygous for the mutant gene.

DNA analysis

DNA can be extracted from any nucleated tissue sample, including blood leucocytes, buccal mucosal cells, skin fibroblasts, amniotic fluid cells and chorionic villus samples. A 10-ml blood sample anticoagulated with EDTA (ethylenediamine tetra-acetic acid) should be maintained at ambient temperature. Once extracted, the DNA is stored frozen, in which state it is stable and available for future analysis for many years. This can be particularly important for lethal inherited conditions as, for some, a test is not yet available or a test might only be required in the future long after the affected person(s) in the family has died. DNA can be extracted from stored pathological material (e.g. paraffin blocks) but the quality is not as good as from a fresh sample.

Mutations of DNA are divided into length mutations with gain or loss of DNA and point mutations, which alter the genetic code at a single base.

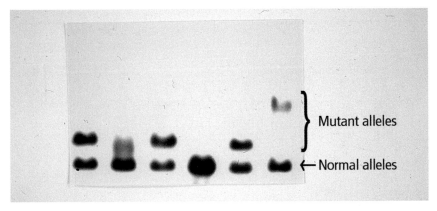

Figure 1.23 DNA analysis for the myotonic dystrophy gene

In all point mutations and most length mutations the mutation is stable and each affected person in the family will have an identical mutation. In some disorders caused by length mutations, the mutation is unstable and varies in size between family members. Figure 1.23 shows an example of DNA analysis for an unstable length mutation in the gene for myotonic dystrophy (an autosomal dominant form of muscular dystrophy). DNA samples from each person have been fragmented and run on an electrophoresis gel. Smaller fragments migrate furthest and specific fragments from the myotonic dystrophy gene have been identified with a gene probe. The normal person has a dense single band that represents DNA sequences from both chromosomal copies of the normal gene. In contrast, each affected person has two bands of lower density representing DNA sequences from the normal and mutant alleles. The mutant alleles are larger and so travel more slowly through the gel. In this family, the affected members show mutations of different sizes.

Figures 1.24–1.26 show an example of a stable three-base pair deletion in the gene for cystic fibrosis. A DNA fragment surrounding the mutation has been visualised by the creation of thousands of copies using the polymerase chain reaction (PCR). Samples from each person are then run on a DNA sequencer to provide accurate sizing. In Figure 1.24, the person is a carrier for cystic fibrosis with one peak for the normal gene (F508) and one for the 3bp deletion (delF508). In Figure 1.25, the person is homozygous for the normal gene (with a single enlarged peak in this position) and in Figure 1.26 the person is homozygous for the mutant gene (with a single enlarged peak in this position). This type of analysis can be used, as in this example, to simultaneously screen for multiple specific mutations in the same gene.

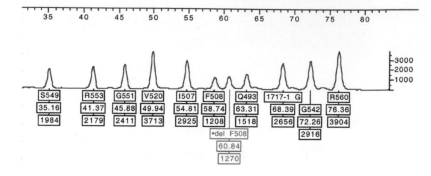

Figure 1.24 DNA analysis for the cystic fibrosis gene

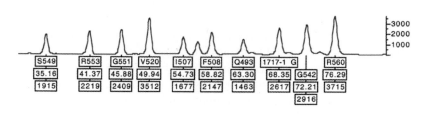

Figure 1.25 DNA analysis for the cystic fibrosis gene

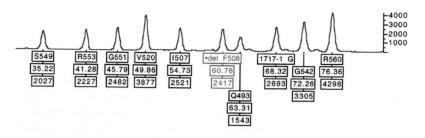

Figure 1.26 DNA analysis for the cystic fibrosis gene

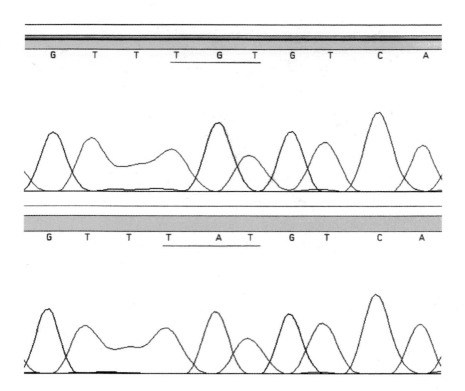

Figure 1.27 DNA analysis for the *HPRT* gene

Figures 1.27 and 1.28 show an example of a stable point mutation in the *HPRT* gene, which causes Lesch–Nyhan syndrome. DNA sequence of the affected region of the gene is shown for each person, with coloured peaks representing each base in the sense strand of DNA, with normal sequence in the upper section and sample sequence in the lower section. The mutation in the affected boy in Figure 1.27 is the substitution of an A for a G. His mother (Figure 1.28) is a carrier with a G representing the normal *HPRT* gene and a superimposed A representing the mutant gene.

Once the molecular basis of the disease is known in a family, it can be used to identify other family members at risk and to provide prenatal diagnosis for serious conditions or presymptomatic testing (Table 1.3).

DNA testing is now available for many single-gene disorders (Table 1.3). For the current situation regarding a particular condition, see Appendix 1, which gives sources of genetic information, including web-based resources that are continually updated.

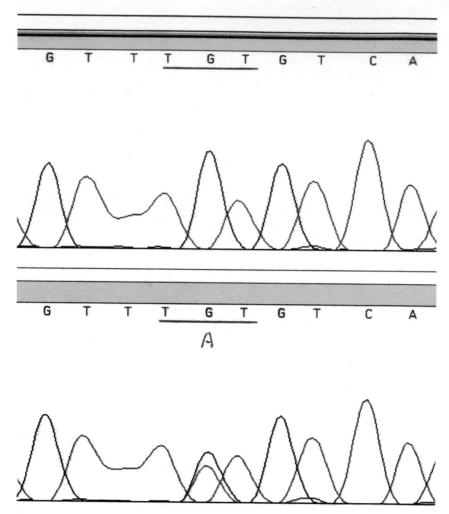

Figure 1.28 DNA analysis for the *HPRT* gene

Chromosome analysis

Chromosomes can be seen with a light microscope in any dividing tissue. In clinical practice, they are most commonly studied in peripheral blood lymphocytes, amniotic fluid cells, chorionic villus samples, bone marrow samples and cultured skin fibroblasts (Box 1.1).

Cells are stimulated to divide and are then arrested in mid-division. The cell membranes are ruptured, releasing the nuclei and a small

Table 1.3 Indications for DNA analysis

Time of DNA analysis	Indications
Prenatally	Diagnosis of at-risk pregnancy (e.g. family history of Duchenne muscular dystrophy)
Neonatally	Confirmation of diagnosis (e.g. cystic fibrosis detected by newborn screening)
Children	Investigation of learning disabilities (exclusion of fragile X syndrome) Confirmation of diagnosis of a childhood-onset disorder (e.g. Duchenne muscular dystrophy)
Adults	Carrier testing (e.g. family history of cystic fibrosis) Presymptomatic testing (e.g. family history of ovarian cancer) Confirmation of diagnosis of adult-onset disorder (e.g. Huntington's disease)

volume of the suspension of nuclei is dropped on to a microscope slide. This ruptures the nuclear membrane and the chromosomes spread out on the slide (Figure 1.29). The magnified (1000x) image of the chromosomes from a single cell is photographed or captured electronically for karyotype analysis.

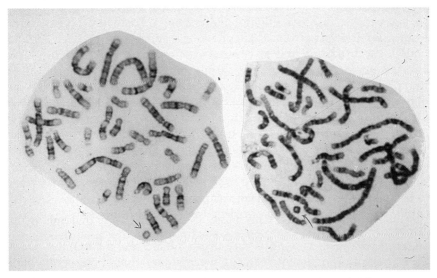

Figure 1.29 Chromosome analysis (an additional chromosomal fragment is arrowed)

BOX 1·1. INDICATIONS FOR CHROMOSOME ANALYSIS

Prenatal chromosome analysis:

- Elevated screening risk of Down syndrome
- Parent with a balanced chromosomal translocation
- Previous child with Down syndrome or other autosomal trisomy

Chromosome analysis in neonates:

- Investigation of multiple malformations
- Confirmation of clinical diagnosis (e.g. Down syndrome)

Chromosome analysis in children:

- Investigation of learning disabilities

Chromosome analysis in adults:

- Investigation of female or male infertility
- Investigation of recurrent miscarriages
- Family members at risk of carrying a balanced translocation

Referral for genetic assessment and counselling

When a patient asks for genetic advice or if a healthcare professional suggests that a disorder might have a genetic basis and seeks advice from a medical geneticist about diagnosis and genetic advice for the family, the usual method of communication is by referral letter. The affected person who brings the family to medical attention is called the 'proband' and the person who is seeking advice, and who may or may not be affected, is called the 'consultand'. Contact details for the UK network of regional genetics centres are provided at the web address: www.bshg.org.uk/Directory/UKdirectory.htm.

When a family is seen at the genetic clinic a detailed family tree is drawn and the diagnosis is confirmed in each affected person. Depending on the condition, genetic tests may need to be performed or the patient may need to be referred to another specialist. Apparently healthy members of the family may need to be examined in case they show mild signs of the disorder.

Genetic disorders may affect any organ system and a condition might have multiple component features. Recognition that these component features are interlinked (that is, they are a syndrome) is crucial for clinical management. Problems can arise when individual specialists concentrate on single components and no one sees the whole picture. The process is not helped by the variability of many syndromes. The classic textbook descriptions are uncommon and most patients do not have a 'full house' of clinical features.

Genetic counselling will cover all aspects of the condition including the prognosis for affected persons, carrier risks for healthy persons, recurrence risks and reproductive options. Accurate diagnosis is of paramount importance for meaningful genetic counselling, so counselling should never precede the steps involved in diagnosis as outlined above. Ideally, both parents should be counselled and adequate time allowed in an appropriate setting. Few couples can be counselled in less than 30 minutes and neither the corner of a hospital ward nor a crowded clinic room is adequate. It is inappropriate to counsel too soon after bereavement or after the initial shock of a serious diagnosis. The depth of explanation needs to be matched to the educational background of the couple and compared with other information they have gleaned from medical sources, parent support groups and internet sites. Counselling must be non-judgemental and nondirective. The aim is to deliver a balanced version of the facts that will permit those who are seeking advice to reach their own decisions with regard to their reproductive future.

BOX 1·2. COMMON MISCONCEPTIONS ABOUT HEREDITY

- Absence of other affected family members means that a disorder present in only one person is not genetic.
- Presence of other affected family members means that a disorder is always genetic.
- If only males or females are affected in the family then only this sex can be affected.
- Any condition present at birth (i.e. congenital) must be genetic.
- Upsets, mental and physical, of the mother in pregnancy cause malformations.
- A one in four risk means that the next three children will be unaffected.
- Confusion of odds, fractions and percentage risks.
- All genetic disorders and their carrier state can be detected by chromosomal analysis.
- All genetic disorders and their carrier state can be detected by DNA analysis.

The pedigree number is the same for all members of a family and each person's records are stored in the family case notes that are indexed under this number. This facilitates interpretation of the family tree and the results of any genetic tests. It also makes it easier to ensure that all at-risk family members have been offered genetic advice. Although many families choose to come to the clinic as a group, the principles of medical confidentiality should still be observed. Many people would not wish relatives to know the results of their genetic tests. Following the consultation a letter summarising the information is sent to the consultands with copies to the referring clinician and the consultand's general practitioner. A medical version of the same information is also sent to the referring clinician and the consultand's general practitioner.

Consultands often feel guilty or stigmatised and it is important to recognise and allay this. Common misconceptions about heredity may also need to be dispelled (Box 1.2).

For certain conditions, such as balanced translocations, autosomal dominant traits and X-linked recessive traits, an extended family study will be required and it is useful to enlist the aid of the consultands in approaching other family members at risk.

Many consultands can be fully counselled at one sitting, but some will require follow-up sessions. If new opportunities arise (such as an improved carrier or prenatal diagnostic test) consultands can be contacted and offered a return appointment.

Section Two

Common genetic problems in obstetric and gynaecological practice

Common genetic problems in obstetric and gynaecological practice

Introduction

This section highlights the common situations in obstetric and gynaecological practice where there are genetic implications.

Genetic causes of infertility

About one in ten couples is involuntarily infertile. Investigation of both male and female primary infertility should include chromosome analysis. An additional investigation in the male is DNA testing for milder combinations of cystic fibrosis mutations. These result in absence of the vas deferens and infertility but no other features of cystic fibrosis.

One of the most common chromosomal causes of male infertility is Klinefelter syndrome, which is usually not diagnosed until adulthood. In addition to infertility, patients may show mild undermasculinisation and gynaecomastia. Intelligence and general lifespan are usually within the normal range. There is an increased risk (7%) of diabetes mellitus and male breast cancer. Management will include assessment for hormonal replacement and screening for complications.

The diagnosis of Klinefelter syndrome is established by chromosome analysis, which reveals 47 chromosomes in total with an additional X chromosome (Figure 2.1). Despite hormone replacement, men with Klinefelter syndrome are infertile and so there is not a genetic implication for their offspring.

One of the most common chromosomal causes of primary female infertility is Turner syndrome. The diagnosis of Turner syndrome is established by chromosomal analysis. This usually reveals only 45 chromosomes in total, with a single X chromosome (see Figure 1.6). There are several other less common chromosomal patterns that also result in Turner syndrome.

The frequency of Turner syndrome at conception is estimated to be as high as 1%. The majority of these pregnancies spontaneously miscarry and most are undiagnosed. Clinical suspicion during pregnancy may be raised by the ultrasound appearance with nuchal oedema in a female fetus (Figure 2.2). Surviving fetuses may occasionally be diagnosed in the

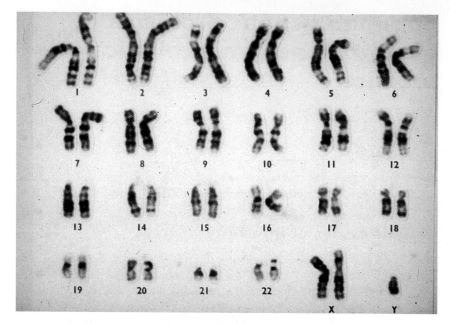

Figure 2.1 Karyotype of Klinefelter syndrome: 47,XXY

newborn period if they show the combination of puffy hands and feet, deepset nails and neck webbing (Figure 2.3) but most remain undiagnosed until they are investigated for childhood short stature or adult infertility. The classic depiction of an adult with Turner syndrome with marked neck webbing, a broad chest and a wide elbow-carrying angle relates to only a minority of women and many are normal apart from short stature and infertility. Intelligence is normal. Short stature is universal, with an untreated adult height of about 1.5 m. Infertility is usual but not invariable and 10% have a spontaneous menarche. Women with Turner syndrome have an increased risk of congenital heart disease, especially coarctation of the aorta and of systemic hypertension.

Management of women with Turner syndrome includes childhood use of growth promoting agents and replacement of female sex hormones.

Genetic causes of recurrent miscarriages

At least one in six recognised pregnancies ends as a miscarriage and so, by chance alone, several miscarriages are not uncommon. Genetic investigation is appropriate for three or more unexplained first-trimester miscarriages as, in this situation, one parent will be found to be a carrier of a chromosomal translocation in 5% of investigated couples.

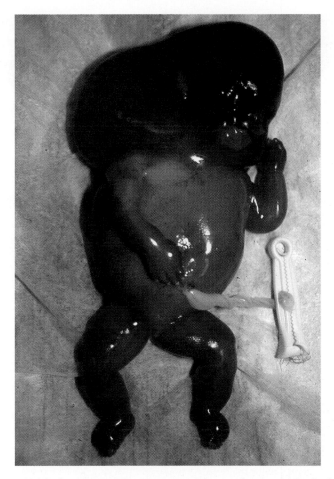

Figure 2.2 Nuchal oedema in a Turner syndrome fetus which died *in utero*

In the family shown in Figure 2.4, the couple was investigated in view of their recurrent miscarriages. Parental chromosomes revealed a normal karyotype in the father but the mother had a translocation between chromosomes 8 and 9 (Figure 2.5). Genetic counselling of these parents would cover how the translocation arose, its implications for the carrier's health, its implications for the next pregnancy and its implications for other family members. When chromosomes break, the ends are sticky and normally reunite with no clinical effect. If, however, more than two chromosomes break at the same time there is a chance that the sticky ends will unite in a new arrangement. For this family, breaks have occurred in

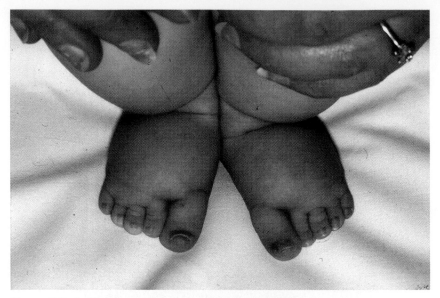

Figure 2.3 Puffy feet in a neonate with Turner syndrome

chromosomes 8 and 9, either at the time the mother was conceived or in an earlier generation. Generally, genes are not damaged at the chromosomal breakpoints and they function normally despite the new arrangement. This is termed a balanced translocation, as the carrier has no loss or gain of genetic material. The carrier mother can thus be reassured that the fact that she is a carrier of a translocation will not influence her general health or lifespan.

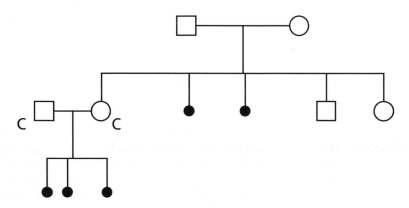

Figure 2.4 Pedigree showing recurrent miscarriages

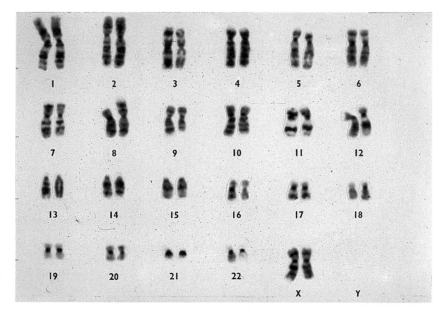

Figure 2.5 Karyotype with a balanced translocation between chromosomes 8 and 9

The genetic implications for this mother relate to reproduction. Her partner passes on one copy of chromosome 8 and one of chromosome 9. She must pass either the normal copy or the translocated copy of each chromosome (Figure 2.6). She can thus have children with normal chromosomes, children with the same balanced translocation as herself and children with various gains or losses of chromosomal material. These gains or losses may result in an early spontaneous miscarriage but this is not invariable and a liveborn child with such an imbalance would have multiple congenital malformations and major learning difficulties. The overall additional risk for this couple (or any couple where a translocation is identified during the investigation of recurrent miscarriages) of having a liveborn disabled child is 5% and prenatal diagnosis and chromosome analysis needs to be discussed. The couple will need to consider the relative advantages and disadvantages of chorionic villus sampling (CVS) and amniocentesis. Amniocentesis is generally performed from 16 weeks of gestation onwards and a result is usually available in 2 weeks. In consequence, couples faced with a serious chromosomal imbalance in the fetus need to consider a late termination of pregnancy. CVS can be offered from 10 weeks of pregnancy and usually gives a more rapid result than amniocentesis. Hence, if requested, a first-trimester termination of pregnancy is possible. The disadvantages of CVS are its restricted availability

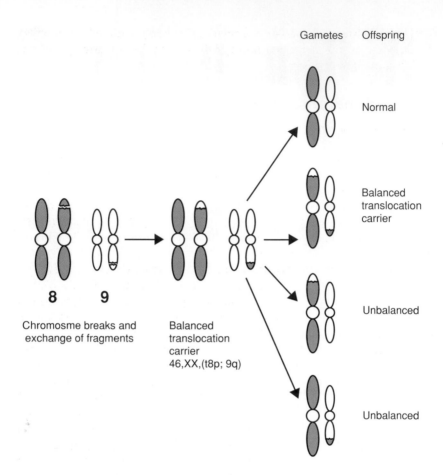

Gametes   Offspring

Normal

Balanced
translocation
carrier

Unbalanced

Unbalanced

8   9

Chromosme breaks and
exchange of fragments

Balanced
translocation
carrier
46,XX,(t8p; 9q)

Figure 2.6 Types of gametes for a carrier of an 8;9 chromosomal
translocation

and the fact that the test itself carries a higher risk of miscarriage. This risk
is commonly quoted as 4%, which means that, for every 100 tests, four
pregnancies are lost. For amniocentesis, the commonly quoted risk of
miscarriage due to the procedure is 1%.

As for other genetic disorders, the medical responsibility of the clinician
who makes the diagnosis relates to the whole family and not just one
patient. In the family shown in Figure 2.4, the first step is to offer to test
the mother's parents' chromosomes. If these are normal then the
translocation has arisen at the time the mother was conceived and risks to
other family members will be very low. In this family, the mother's father
was found to carry the same balanced translocation and testing of her

brother and sister and the father's relatives should be offered. In practice, investigation of the extended family will usually be undertaken by the local regional genetics service.[1]

Elevated maternal screening risk

DOWN SYNDROME

In the absence of a family history, the risk of Down syndrome in a pregnancy can be calculated from a combination of the mother's age and the results of biophysical tests.

The risk or probability of an event ranges from one (100% or always happens) to zero (0% or never happens). On the basis of maternal age alone, the risk of Down syndrome at birth varies from one in 1500 for a 20-year-old mother to one in 28 for a 45-year-old mother (Table 2.1).

In the second trimester, analysis of maternal biochemical markers, a variable combination of free beta human chorionic gonadotrophin (FβhCG), total human chorionic gonadotrophin (hCG), alphafetoprotein (α-FP) and unconjugated oestriol, can also provide a relative risk figure for the presence of Down syndrome in that pregnancy.

These risks, from maternal age and maternal biochemistry, are independent of each other and can thus be combined by multiplication. For example, from Table 2.1, a 30-year-old mother has an age-related risk of one in 900. Her level of αFP is 0.7 multiples of the median (MOM) and this gives a likelihood ratio (relative heights of the two curves) of 1.5 (Figure 2.7). Her level of hCG is 2.6 MOM and this gives a likelihood ratio of 3.0 (Figure 2.8). These biochemical markers are independent of each other and of maternal age so the risks are combined by multiplication. Her combined risk is thus one in 200 (1:900 × 3:1 × 1.5:1.0). The level of risk

Table 2.1 Frequency of Down syndrome at birth in relation to maternal age	
Maternal age (years)	Frequency of Down syndrome at birth
20	1:1500
25	1:1350
30	1:900
35	1:380
37	1:240
39	1:150
41	1:85
43	1:50
45	1:28

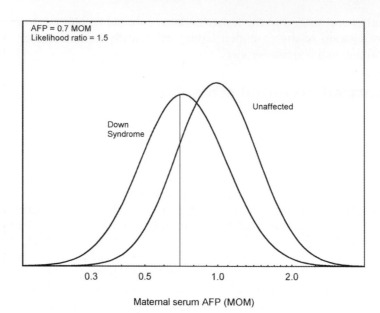

Figure 2.7 Use of maternal serum α-FP expressed in multiples of the median to give a likelihood ratio for Down syndrome in the second trimester

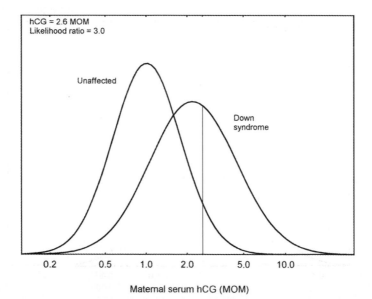

Figure 2.8 Use of maternal serum hCG expressed in multiples of the median to give a likelihood ratio for Down syndrome in the second trimester

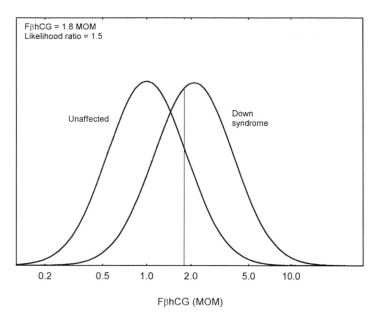

Figure 2.9 Use of maternal serum FβhCG expressed in multiples of the median to give a likelihood ratio for Down syndrome in the first trimester

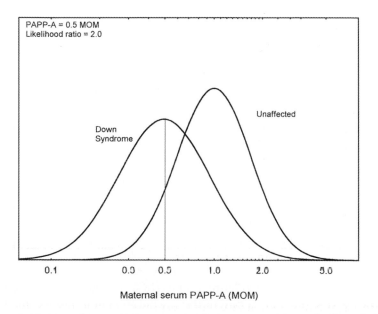

Figure 2.10 Use of maternal serum PAPP-A expressed in multiples of the median to give a likelihood ratio for Down syndrome in the first trimester

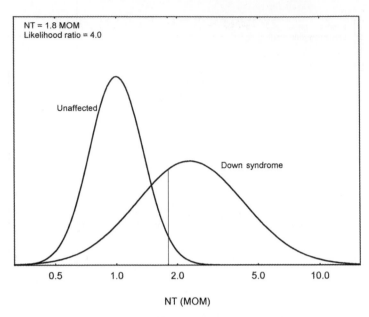

NT = 1.8 MOM
Likelihood ratio = 4.0

Unaffected

Down syndrome

0.5   1.0   2.0   5.0   10.0

NT (MOM)

Figure 2.11 Use of sagittal thickness of the nuchal fold expressed in multiples of the median to give a likelihood ratio for Down syndrome in the first trimester

at which an amniocentesis is offered varies but is commonly one in 250 or higher. Thus, this woman would fall in the high-risk category and be eligible for prenatal chromosome analysis.

In the first-trimester analysis of maternal biochemical markers (usually a combination of FβhCG and pregnancy-associated plasma protein A, (PAPP-A) can also provide a relative risk figure for the presence of Down syndrome in that pregnancy. This can be combined with the maternal age-related risk (from Table 2.1) and with a further independent risk based on the sagittal thickness of the nuchal fold (nuchal translucency) on ultrasound examination.

As these three risks in the first trimester are independent of each other, again they can be combined by multiplication. For example, a 30-year-old mother has an age-related risk at birth of one in 900. Her level of FβhCG is 1.8 MOM and this gives a likelihood ratio of 1.5 (Figure 2.9). Her level of PAPP-A is 0.5 MOM and this gives a likelihood ratio of 2.0 (Figure 2.10). Her fetal nuchal thickness measurement is 1.8 MOM and this gives a likelihood ratio of 4.0 (Figure 2.11). These biochemical markers are independent of each other and of the nuchal thickness and the maternal age and so are combined by multiplication. Her combined risk is thus one in 75 (1:900 × 1.5:1 × 2:1 × 4:1).

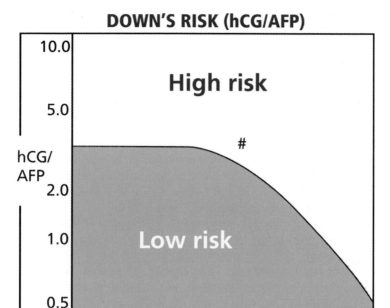

DOWN'S RISK (hCG/AFP)

High risk

Low risk

hCG/AFP

Maternal age (Years)

Figure 2.12 Combined risk reported as a diagram with a threshold between high risk and low risk

In communication of these risks to the patient, several difficulties need to be anticipated and covered. First, this is a screening test and not a diagnostic test. A diagnostic test confirms or refutes a diagnosis in an individual and should be 100% reliable. In contrast, a screening test aims to identify high- and low-risk groups and has to be the first step when universal use of the diagnostic test is impractical. The high-risk group will contain most but not all affected pregnancies but will also include many normal pregnancies. The low-risk group will still contain some affected pregnancies but most will be normal pregnancies. As only those in the high-risk group are offered the diagnostic test (in this case fetal chromosome analysis) not all affected pregnancies can be detected and the sensitivity will be less than 100%. In second-trimester screening programmes the sensitivity or detection rate is about 70%, which means that the false negative rate is about 30%. In first-trimester screening the sensitivity or detection rate is 90%.

The overall chance that a woman who has a screening test will be offered a diagnostic test is one in 20. If a woman then has a diagnostic test, the overall chance of finding Down syndrome is one in 45 with second-trimester screening and one in 30 with first-trimester screening.

The second difficulty relates to understanding risks. Some people fully understand the meaning of a one in 100 risk but many need further explanation with, for example, alternative expressions as percentages or as odds of normality (e.g. 99 times out of 100 will be normal). It may also be helpful to translate risks into revised maternal age risks. Thus a 40-year-old mother with a combined risk of one in 380 equates to that for a 35-year-old mother and she may decide against fetal chromosome analysis. Some people may find it helpful to see how close they are to the threshold between high and low risk (Figure 2.12).

The third difficulty relates to the parents' perception of Down syndrome. Maternal screening is only appropriate in the absence of a family history of Down syndrome and the parents will thus have little or no direct knowledge about the condition. The main problem for children with Down syndrome relates to major learning difficulties. Typically, children will learn to walk and talk but will remain dependent on their parents or carers. They have minor physical characteristics that aid clinical diagnosis. About one-third will have major congenital heart malformations that may need surgical correction. In the absence of congenital heart disease or with successful correction, the average life span is still reduced because of other complications including dementia and leukaemia (1%).

It is essential that parents offered antenatal screening programmes should have adequate information about the condition and the limitations of the test in order to make an informed choice.

NEURAL TUBE DEFECT

In the absence of a family history of a neural tube defect (anencephaly, spina bifida or encephalocele), the risk for a pregnancy can be assessed by maternal serum screening. Open neural tube defects lack a covering of skin over the lesion and fetal α-FP can thus leak into the amniotic fluid and then reach the maternal circulation. In normal pregnancies, maternal serum α-FP (MSα-FP) levels start to rise from 10 weeks and peak at around 32 weeks before falling to term. First-trimester screening for neural tube defects using MSα-FP is not possible, as the levels are not elevated until mid-pregnancy. Thus, measurement of MSα-FP is undertaken at 15–20 (optimum 16–17) completed weeks of gestation (Figure 2.13). If the level is above the 95th centile (equivalent to two MOM for that gestation), detailed fetal ultrasound is indicated, as there is a 2% chance of a neural tube defect.

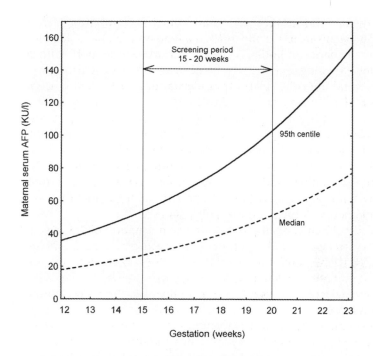

Figure 2.13 Maternal serum α-FP centiles for the screening period

As emphasised for Down syndrome screening, several difficulties need to be anticipated and covered in communication with the parent. First, this is a screening programme that aims to identify a high-risk group who can then be offered the diagnostic test for a neural tube defect (detailed ultrasound scanning). The sensitivity or detection rate depends on the type of defect. Anencephaly (Figure 2.14) is always 'open', with no skin covering, and the area of exposed tissue gives extremely high levels of MSα-FP. The sensitivity is thus virtually 100% for anencephaly. Spina bifida is 'open' in 80–85% of cases (Figure 2.15). The 'closed' skin-covered lesions (Figure 2.16) cannot be detected using this method of screening. The size of open spina bifida varies from extensive lesions that can cause elevations of MSα-FP similar to those seen for anencephalic pregnancies to small lesions, which may not produce abnormal elevations of MSα-FP. The sensitivity of MSα-FP screening for open spina bifida is 88%. Thus, 12% of open spina bifida will be assigned to the low-risk group and missed.

The second difficulty relates to understanding risk figures. The overall risk for the high-risk group of having a neural tube defect is one in 50 but, in practice, numerical risks are usually avoided and the mother is assigned

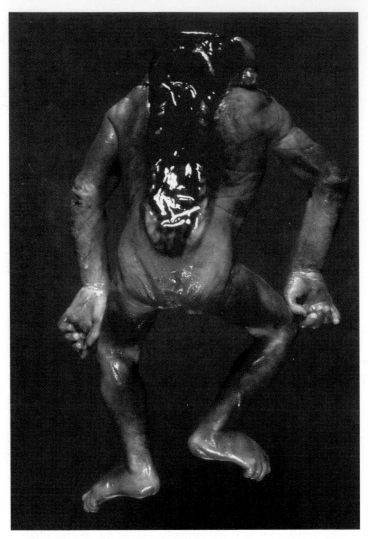

Figure 2.14 Anencephaly and extensive open spina bifida

as high risk or low risk. We also provide this information in pictorial form, as it helps parents who are close to the borderline between high and low risk to make decisions about further testing (figure 2.12).

The third difficulty relates to providing the couple with an outlook for the affected pregnancy. Stillbirth or neonatal death is invariable for anencephaly but the prognosis for spina bifida is more difficult to predict.

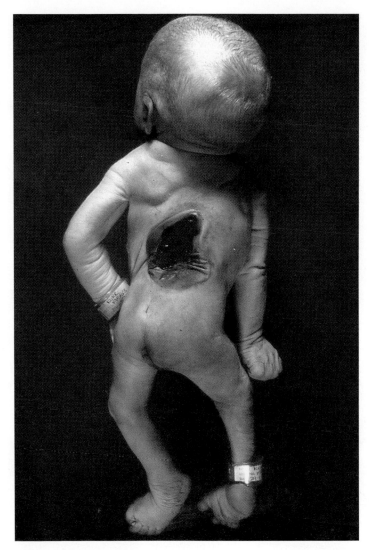

Figure 2.15 Open spina bifida

With surgery within 24 hours for open spina bifida, 40% survive more than 7 years but only 8% have little or no disability, 10% are moderately disabled and 82% severely disabled. Babies with gross paralysis of the legs, thoracolumbar or thoracolumbar–sacral lesions, kyphoscoliosis, hydrocephalus at birth or associated abnormalities have a particularly poor

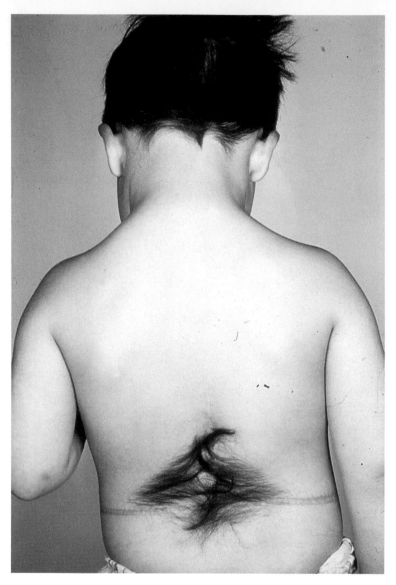

Figure 2.16 Closed spina bifida

prognosis. In contrast, 60% of babies with closed lesions survive to 5 years and one-third are free of disability, with one-third moderately disabled and one-third severely disabled.

It is essential that women offered antenatal screening programmes should have adequate information about the condition and the limitations of the test in order to make an informed choice.

CYSTIC FIBROSIS

Cystic fibrosis is a relatively common cause of childhood morbidity and mortality. The clinical severity is variable, with problems mainly relating to pancreatic insufficiency and chronic lung disease secondary to recurrent infection. The median survival despite early diagnosis and advances in treatment is currently 25 years.

One in 2000 pregnancies is affected. Affected pregnancies can be identified by screening both parents for cystic fibrosis carrier status. The affected pregnancies have inherited an underactive *CFTR* gene from each parent. The parents are carriers (heterozygous) with one normal *CFTR* gene on one copy of chromosome 7 and one underactive *CFTR* gene on the opposite copy of chromosome 7. For these carrier parents, on average one in four of their pregnancies will inherit two copies of the underactive cystic fibrosis gene (see Figure 1.12, autosomal recessive inheritance).

Over 500 different types of mutation in the *CFTR* gene have been described. One, a three-base deletion at position 508 (delF508 or ΔF508), is the single most common mutation (see Figures 1.24–1.26). This mutation accounts for 70–80% of the underactive *CFTR* alleles in northern Europe and the USA but is less common in southern Europe (45–55%), African Americans (37%) and Ashkenazi Jews (30%). Most of the other mutations are individually uncommon, with occasional exceptions in association with particular ethnic groups (such as W1282X, which accounts for 48% of mutant *CFTR* alleles in Ashkenazi Jews).

This wide variety of *CFTR* mutations means that it is not practicable to exclude all known mutations in screening for cystic fibrosis carrier status. In practice, a panel of common mutations is tested, which identifies nearly 90% of *CFTR* mutations in northern European populations. In screening programmes, mouthwash samples for DNA analysis are collected from the pregnant woman and her partner. Her sample is tested with the panel of mutations and if it is found to be positive his sample is then tested. If his sample is also positive the pregnancy has a one in four risk of being affected and the couple can opt for prenatal diagnosis by fetal DNA analysis.

This type of screening does not test for all known cystic fibrosis mutations and thus there is a residual risk even if either partner tests negative.

When either or both parents are found to be carriers of cystic fibrosis, there is also a need to consider extended family testing for carrier status.

Family history

DOWN SYNDROME

Most (95%) cases of Down syndrome are caused by an extra free copy of chromosome 21, resulting in 47 chromosomes in total, with three copies of chromosome 21 (trisomy 21, see Figure 1.3). In this situation, the parental karyotypes will be normal and the risk of recurrence for the parents of trisomy 21 or other major chromosomal abnormality at amniocentesis is 1.5% (risk at birth 1%). This risk is added to the mother's age-related risk (Table 2.1). Thus, for example, the recurrence risk at birth for a 43-year-old mother with a previous child with trisomy 21 is 3% (one in 50 added to 1%).

In this situation, the risks are added rather than multiplied. In earlier examples risks were multiplied together as they represented independent risks (such as the risk of Down syndrome on the basis of maternal age and the relative risk of Down syndrome based on maternal biochemistry). Mutually exclusive risks are added. These can be spotted by the use of words like 'either' and 'or'. Hence, for this example with a recurrence of trisomy 21, the pregnancy may be affected either as a result of maternal age or as a result of the previous affected child but cannot have trisomy 21 twice over.

Hence, for parents with a previous child or pregnancy affected by trisomy 21, there is a recurrence risk, which is higher than the population risk and many couples will seek reassurance by fetal chromosome analysis in future pregnancies. In this situation, the risks are not increased for other relatives above the general population risks and no special testing is indicated either before or during pregnancies. These relatives would not require blood karyotyping and would be offered routine antenatal screening tests for Down syndrome.

An important minority (5%) of cases of Down syndrome are caused by chromosome translocations involving chromosome 21. The clinical features of translocation Down syndrome are indistinguishable from those due to trisomy 21 and karyotyping is required to establish the diagnosis. The karyotype of a patient with translocation Down syndrome is shown in Figure 2.17. This patient has 46 chromosomes in total, with two free copies of chromosome 21 and one extra copy of 21, which is joined to the top of chromosome 14. This translocation between chromosomes 14 and 21 might have occurred as a new event at the time the egg or sperm was produced or it might have been inherited. Hence, the parental karyotypes of a child or pregnancy with translocation Down syndrome must be examined. In this family, the mother's karyotype was normal but the father was found to have the translocation (Figure 2.18). He has only 45 chromosomes in total rather than the normal 46, as two free copies of 14

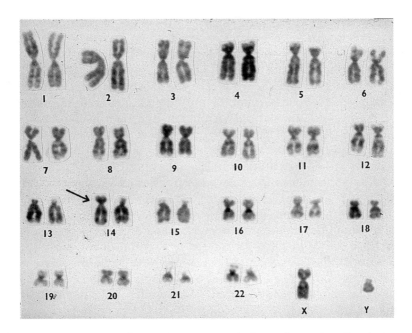

Figure 2.17 Down syndrome due to an unbalanced translocation between chromosomes 14 and 21 (arrowed; chromosomes shown unbanded)

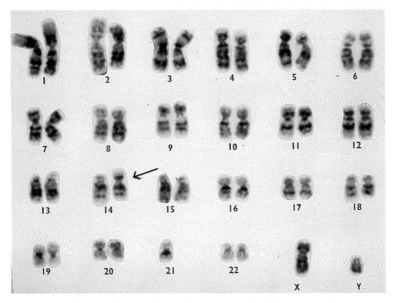

Figure 2.18 Father with a balanced translocation between chromosomes 14 and 21 (arrowed)

and 21 are replaced by a fused single chromosome. In this translocation, he has not lost or gained vital genetic material and hence he has no clinical features and is a balanced translocation carrier. The problem occurs when he comes to hand on chromosomes to a pregnancy. Each sperm must receive one of each pair of chromosomes and this can result in sperm with either normal chromosomes, balanced translocation chromosomes or unbalanced arrangements with gain or loss of chromosomal material (Figure 2.19).

From Figure 2.19, it might be expected that two of every four pregnancies would be chromosomally unbalanced but in practice with this translocation (and with many other translocations) there is selection against sperm (or eggs) with an imbalance and the frequency of unbalanced arrangements at the time of amniocentesis is 1% if the father is the carrier of the balanced translocation and 15% if the mother is the carrier. The couple needs to be offered fetal chromosome analysis after either chorionic villus sampling or amniocentesis in future pregnancies. The relative advantages and disadvantages of each will need to be discussed as outlined in the section on genetic causes of recurrent miscarriage in Section 2.

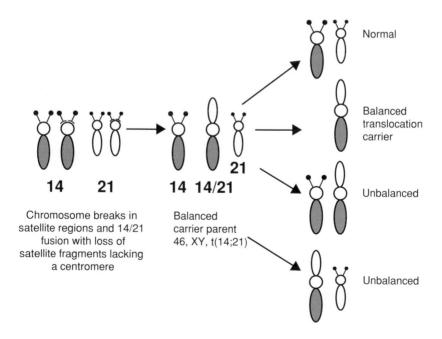

Figure 2.19 Types of gametes for a carrier of a 14;21 chromosomal translocation

Table 2.2 Risks of chromosomally unbalanced offspring for carriers of balanced translocations involving chromosome 21

Translocation	Carrier	Risk of unbalanced arrangement at amniocentesis (%)
14–21	Father	1
14–21	Mother	15
21–22	Father	5
21–22	Mother	10
21–21	Either parent	100

In counselling the family with a chromosomal translocation, the clinical responsibility relates to the whole family. Thus, it is crucial to determine who else in the family also carries a balanced translocation. This can involve extended family studies and is usually undertaken by the regional genetics service.[1]

Translocations involving chromosome 21 can also involve other chromosomes and the risks to offspring depend not only on which chromosomes are involved but also on which parent is the carrier of the balanced translocation (Table 2.2).

In Figure 2.20, the woman is expecting her first child and, at booking, is noted to have a brother with Down syndrome. She does not know whether he ever had a chromosome test and is anxious about an increased risk for Down syndrome in her pregnancy.

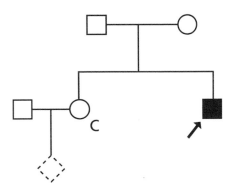

Figure 2.20 Family history of Down syndrome

This is a common situation and the key is to try and discover whether or not her affected brother has trisomy 21 (in which case she can be reassured, given the general population risk and offered routine Down syndrome screening) or has translocation Down syndrome (in which case, further testing in the family is required).

The affected brother's full name, date of birth and addresses (at birth, early childhood and current) are helpful. The genetics centre local to the affected brother should be contacted.[1] The genetics centre should be able to confirm whether or not he has been tested and whether or not he has a translocation or trisomy 21. If no record of testing is found then it would be usual to offer the woman an urgent blood chromosome analysis to exclude a balanced translocation in her and the local genetics centre would undertake to organise testing on the affected brother and other relatives, as required. The alternative of testing the brother first and then only testing the woman if a translocation is found is usually impractical, given the timescale and potential timing of prenatal testing if she is found to be at risk.

NEURAL TUBE DEFECT

The neural groove appears at 20 days from conception; it is mainly closed by 23 days and fully closed by 28 days. Defective closure of the neural tube may occur at any level. Failure at the cephalic end produces anencephaly (Figure 2.14) or encephalocele (Figure 2.21), and failure lower down produces spina bifida (Figures 2.15 and 2.16). Overall, anencephaly (with or without spina bifida) accounts for 40% of neural tube defects, spina bifida alone for 55% and encephalocele for 5%. Other malformations, particularly exomphalos and renal malformations, coexist in 25%.

The frequency of neural tube defects shows geographical and secular variation. In the USA, Africa and Mongolia, one in 1000 births are affected. In southeast England in the 1970s, three in 1000 births were affected and at that time the frequency was even higher (five to eight in 1000) in Ireland, Wales and the West of Scotland. Subsequently, the frequency has fallen throughout the UK and the current figure in the West of Scotland is two in 1000. The reasons for this secular fall are unknown but dietary improvements are believed to be a contributory factor.

Family and twin studies support multifactorial (part-genetic) inheritance for neural tube defects. The genetic components of susceptibility are unknown but one environmental component, maternal levels of folic acid during early pregnancy, has been identified.

In the UK, the recurrence risk for any neural tube defect after an affected pregnancy is one in 25–33 (3–4%) and this risk is reduced to one in 100 by folic acid supplementation, which must be introduced prior to

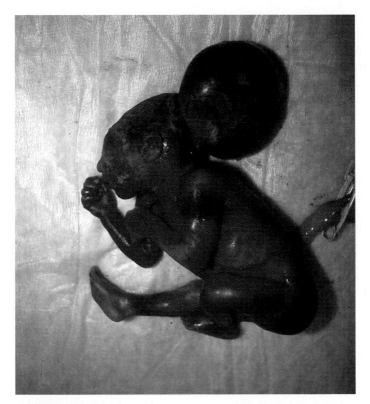

Figure 2.21 Encephalocele

conception at a dosage of 5 mg/day. Prenatal diagnosis can be offered by means of detailed ultrasound scanning. The risk to the offspring of an affected woman is also one in 25–33 (3–4%). If a couple has two or more affected children the recurrence risk rises to one in ten.

For second-degree relatives (aunts/uncles, nephews/nieces) the risk is one in 70 and for third-degree relatives (cousins) it is one in 150.

CYSTIC FIBROSIS

As described above, cystic fibrosis is an important cause of chronic morbidity and mortality in childhood. It is inherited as an autosomal recessive disorder and one in 22 of northern European and US populations are carriers. When two carriers have children, there is on average a one in four chance that they will inherit both copies of the underactive *CFTR* gene and be affected.

A wide variety (over 500) of mutations in the *CFTR* gene have been identified. A 3bp deletion at position 508 (delF508 or ΔF508) is the single most common mutation (see Figures 1.24–1.26). This mutation accounts for 70–80% of mutant cystic fibrosis genes in northern Europe and the USA. Most other mutations are individually uncommon. About 50% of northern European and US patients have two copies of ΔF508 (ΔF508/ΔF508); most of the rest will have one copy of ΔF508 and one other mutant gene (ΔF508/M) and a minority will have two copies of other mutant (M) genes (M/M).

Figure 2.22 shows a family with cystic fibrosis. The woman is expecting her second child and was alarmed to hear that her niece has been diagnosed with cystic fibrosis. Her sister (the mother of the affected girl) must be a carrier of cystic fibrosis, as must her partner. DNA testing confirmed this and also identified that the pregnant woman's mother was a carrier (normal/mutant, N/M). The pregnant woman therefore had a one in two risk of being a carrier and her DNA test confirmed that she had inherited the mutant gene. Her husband is of North European origin and has no family history of the disease and so has the one in 22 general population carrier risk. Before he is tested, the risk to the pregnancy of being affected by cystic fibrosis is one in 88. This represents her chance of passing the mutant allele on (1 × 0.5 – her carrier risk multiplied by 0.5) combined with his chance of passing on the mutant allele (one in 22 × 0.5 – his carrier risk multiplied by 0.5). If testing identifies that he is a carrier, this risk to the pregnancy becomes one in four. If his screen for common cystic fibrosis mutations is negative the risk to the pregnancy will

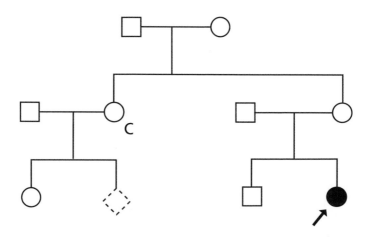

Figure 2.22 Family history of cystic fibrosis

be substantially reduced. (If the cystic fibrosis screen detects 90% of mutations, the residual risk of the disease for the pregnancy will be one in 880 – her carrier risk multiplied by 0.5 multiplied by his residual carrier risk multiplied by 0.5 = 1 × 0.5 × one in 22 × one in ten × 0.5.)

MUSCULAR DYSTROPHY

A family history of muscular dystrophy always needs to be taken seriously. There are many subtypes of muscular dystrophy and most are inherited as single-gene disorders. This means that there are likely to be high recurrence risks for close family members and, for X-linked forms, even quite distant female relatives may still be at high risk. In light of the severity of many of these conditions, parents will commonly request reassurance by means of prenatal diagnosis.

Duchenne muscular dystrophy (DMD) is the most common form of childhood muscular dystrophy, with a birth incidence of one in 3000 males. The gene for DMD is located on the short arm of the X chromosome and so males are always affected, whereas females with a single mutant DMD gene on one X chromosome and a normal copy on the other X chromosome are usually normal. Affected males are normal at birth but already have high levels of muscle enzymes such as creatine phosphokinase (CPK) in their serum. Walking may be delayed and they are rarely able to run properly. Muscle weakness is progressive and most will be chair-bound by 12 years of age. Death from respiratory complications usually occurs at around 20 years of age.

Examination of the DMD gene in affected males usually (70%) shows a deletion of variable size; less commonly, a partial duplication or a point mutation is found. These changes can be used to determine which females in the family are carriers and can also be used for the carriers to offer prenatal diagnosis. If the DMD mutation is not known in the family, carrier risks can be calculated from the mother's position in the pedigree, information from the mother's CPK levels, which are elevated in two-thirds of carriers, and by tracking the at-risk chromosome within the family using DNA markers.

In Figure 2.23, the woman has a family history of DMD. Her brother died of DMD and her sister's son has recently been diagnosed with DMD. The mothers of each affected male must be carriers of the DMD mutation, as the alternative explanation of two new mutations is highly unlikely. The pregnant woman's mother is therefore a carrier and must hand on either her X chromosome with the normal gene or the X chromosome with the DMD mutation. The pregnant woman's risk of being a DMD carrier is thus one in two. The risk that her pregnancy is affected with DMD is one in eight (her carrier risk multiplied by her chance of passing

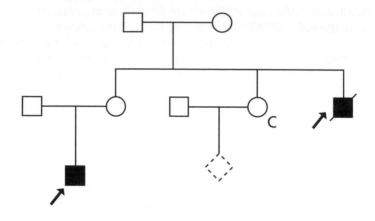

Figure 2.23 Family history of Duchenne muscular dystrophy

on the mutant gene multiplied by the chance of a male pregnancy – one in two × one in two × one in two). If the mutation is known and she is shown to be a carrier this risk rises to one in four and fetal DNA analysis can be used to determine the sex of the fetus and the presence of the DMD mutation. Usually, CVS is the source of the fetal DNA, as this allows the option of a first-trimester termination of pregnancy.

If the mutation in the affected males has not been identified, carrier detection and prenatal diagnosis may still be possible using other methods but will lack 100% accuracy. In this situation, many couples still choose to terminate an at-risk pregnancy because of the severity of the disorder.

Carrier detection within the extended family will be required and every family with DMD should be referred to the regional genetics centre.[1]

Myotonic dystrophy (dystrophia myotonica) is the most common adult onset form of muscular dystrophy, with a frequency of one in 9000. The gene (*DMPK*) for myotonic dystrophy is located on chromosome 19 and the condition is inherited as an autosomal dominant trait. Thus, each affected person has one normal *DMPK* allele and one mutant *DMPK* allele. Unlike most genetic mutations, the *DMPK* mutation is unstable and varies in size in individuals, even in the same family (see Figure 1.23). The mutation tends to increase in size with each generation, particularly when transmitted by the mother. There is an approximate correlation between the size of the mutation and the severity of the condition, with larger mutations causing earlier onset and more severe disability. At the mildest end of the spectrum, there may be few or no symptoms of muscle weakness and perhaps only adult-onset cataracts. More commonly, the affected person has adult-onset progressive muscle weakness, especially of the face, sternomastoids and distal limb muscles. Severe disability is usual 15–20 years from the onset. General anaesthesia may be hazardous and the anaesthetist should be warned of the patient's diagnosis even if there are few or no symptoms. At the most severe end of the spectrum the fetus can be affected. Almost invariably, the mother is the affected parent and the fetus has a *DMPK* allele that is massively expanded. Neonatal hypotonia is marked and these children later show major learning difficulties and progressive muscle weakness. In each of these situations, the clinical diagnosis can be confirmed by DNA analysis. Within a family, presymptomatic testing of healthy at-risk adults and prenatal diagnosis are also possible by DNA analysis.

A significant number of families only come to light following the birth of a severely affected infant. Earlier identification may be possible at the antenatal clinic by recognition of the typical myotonic dystrophy facies with a long thin, expressionless face and ptosis. Sufferers may also demonstrate myotonia, with delayed relaxation after muscle contraction (for instance, after shaking hands).

There are a number of obstetric complications in women with myotonic dystrophy. There may be delay in labour, requiring intervention, and great care must be exercised in using appropriate anaesthetic agents. Postpartum haemorrhage is also common.

There are general medical complications in myotonic dystrophy. These include cardiac rhythm abnormalities and diabetes mellitus, which should be excluded during pregnancy and monitored afterwards.

A pregnant woman with myotonic dystrophy has a one in two risk of transmitting the disorder. Counselling about prenatal diagnosis is difficult because an affected pregnancy may result in either a severely affected neonate or an infant with childhood or adult onset. DNA analysis cannot completely distinguish these outcomes. Delivery of an at-risk child should thus take place in an obstetric unit with an attached neonatal intensive care unit.

In every family, genetic counselling of the extended family will be required and they should be referred to the regional genetics centre.[1]

LEARNING DIFFICULTIES

Moderate and severe learning difficulties (IQ of less than 50) affect 1% of newborns but this figure falls to 0.3–0.4% in children of school age, owing to deaths in infancy from associated abnormalities or rapidly progressive disorders. The cause can be identified in about 75% of these (Table 2.3).

Trisomy 21 is the single most common cause of major learning difficulties in this age group; a variety of other chromosome abnormalities

Table 2.3 Causes of moderate and severe learning difficulties in children of school age

Cause	Occurrence (%)
Chromosomal disorder	
Trisomy 21	25
Other	2
Single gene disorders	
Autosomal dominant	1
Autosomal recessive	10
X-linked	
Fragile X syndrome	4
Other	4
Brain malformations/dysmorphic syndromes[a]	14
Environmental factors	15
Unexplained	25

[a] Excluding recognised chromosomal and single-gene disorders

comprise the other 2%. Over 250 single-gene disorders have been described for which major learning difficulty is a consistent or common feature. Numerically, the most frequent among the autosomal dominant disorders is tuberous sclerosis. Among autosomal recessive disorders, phenylketonuria, cerebral degenerative disorders and recessive microcephaly predominate whereas, among the X-linked disorders, the fragile X syndrome is the single most common cause.

Genetic assessment will thus be directed towards establishing the cause of the disability in the family and referral to the regional genetics centre will be required.[1] When the cause is obscure and no other relatives are affected to suggest a pattern of inheritance, observed (empiric) recurrence risks from the outcome of a large number of similar families need to be used. In the absence of a specific diagnosis, reassurance by prenatal diagnosis during a subsequent pregnancy cannot be offered.

The fragile X syndrome is caused by an unstable length mutation in the *FMR1* gene on the X chromosome. Small increases in length (so-called premutations) of this gene are asymptomatic but, once beyond a critical size, each male will be affected and will show learning difficulties. Females may carry an abnormal gene but are usually, but not always, protected by the presence of a normal-sized gene on the opposite X chromosome. The diagnosis in affected males can be confirmed by DNA analysis and this test can also detect the carriers and be used for prenatal diagnosis.

In Figure 2.24, the consultand has two male cousins with fragile X syndrome. DNA testing revealed that their mother was a carrier and that she had inherited the mutation from her father. He was healthy but had a small premutation (normal transmitting male). As he had to hand on his X chromosome to each daughter, the consultand's mother must be a carrier and the consultand has a one in two risk of being a carrier. The risk to her pregnancy is thus one in eight (her carrier risk multiplied by her chance of passing on the mutant gene multiplied by the chance of a male pregnancy – one in two × one in two × one in two). If she is shown to be a carrier, this risk rises to one in four and fetal DNA analysis can be used to determine the sex of the fetus and the presence of the *FMR1* mutation. Usually CVS is the source of the fetal DNA, as this allows the option of a first-trimester termination of pregnancy.

Carrier detection within the extended family will be required and every family with fragile X syndrome should be referred to the regional genetics centre.[1]

CONGENITAL MALFORMATIONS

Three percent of newborns have a single major congenital malformation and 0.7% of newborns have multiple major malformations. Minor congenital malformations (for example, a single umbilical artery, soft-tissue syndactyly, or ear tags or pits) are even more common and, if multiple, should alert the clinician to the possibility of an associated major

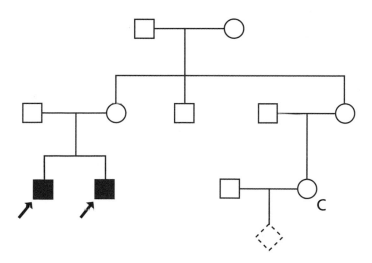

Figure 2.24 Family history of fragile X syndrome

Table 2.4 Aetiology of major congenital malformations

Congenital malformation	Occurence (%)
Idiopathic	60.0
Multifactorial (part-genetic) disorders	20.0
Single-gene disorders	7.5
Chromosomal disorders	6.0
Maternal illness	3.0
Congenital infection	2.0
Drugs, X-rays, alcohol	1.5

malformation. Table 2.4 indicates the identifiable causes of major congenital malformations.

As indicated, the basis of most congenital malformations is unknown. Multifactorial (part-genetic) inheritance is the most common identifiable cause followed by single-gene disorders and chromosomal disorders. Thus, genetic conditions account for at least one-third of all congenital malformations.

Visible duplication of deficiency of any of the autosomes is almost invariably associated with major learning difficulties, postnatal growth deficiency and an unusual facial appearance. Multiple congenital malformations and intrauterine growth restriction are also commonly seen and roughly correlate in severity with the extent of the chromosomal imbalance. Over 250 single-gene disorders include major congenital malformations as a consistent or frequent feature. Recognition of these single-gene disorders and of inherited structural chromosome rearrangements is of clinical importance in view of their potential high recurrence risks.

Maternal illnesses associated with an increased risk of fetal malformation include type 1 (insulin-dependent) diabetes mellitus, epilepsy, alcohol misuse and phenylketonuria. There is a 5–15% risk of congenital malformation (especially congenital heart disease, neural tube defect and sacral agenesis) for the offspring of a diabetic mother in proportion to the quality of her diabetic control (but no increase if the mother has gestational or type 2, non-insulin-dependent, diabetes). The risk is also increased (to about 6%, especially for cleft lip and congenital heart disease) for a mother with epilepsy, although here it is difficult to separate the risk due to the disease and that due to her medication. Untreated maternal phenylketonuria carries a high risk (25%) to the fetus for major learning difficulties, microcephaly and congenital heart disease.

Genetic counselling in families with a family history of congenital malformations will thus depend heavily on identification of the underlying cause. In the absence of an identified cause observed (empiric) recurrence risks derived from the outcome of large numbers of similar families are used. Prenatal diagnosis may be possible using high resolution ultrasound scanning.

OVARIAN CANCER

Ovarian cancer affects 1:50–100 women and familial ovarian cancer accounts for 5–10% of the total. The familial form should be suspected if the woman is young (under 50 years of age), has bilateral disease, has associated tumours or has a relevant family history of ovarian or breast cancer. Non-inherited ovarian cancer has a mean age of onset of 70 years whereas the inherited form often occurs in the 40s and 50s. In non-inherited cancer, mutations cumulate in a clone of cells, which then undergoes malignant transformation. As none of these mutations was inherited, comparable changes are unlikely in the other ovary. In contrast, in the inherited form, the first key genetic mutation is inherited and is present in all cells. This accounts for the earlier age of onset in the inherited form and the increased chance of bilateral involvement.

One of the most common causes of inherited ovarian cancer is familial breast/ovarian cancer. This is inherited as an autosomal dominant trait and in 35–50% of cases is due to mutations in the *BRCA1* gene on the long

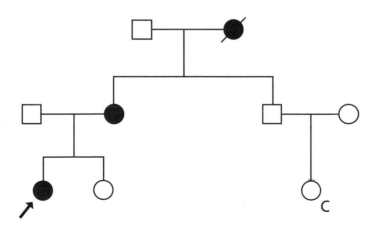

Figure 2.25 Family history of cancer

arm of chromosome 17. For females with a *BRCA1* mutation, the lifetime risk for breast cancer is 80% and for ovarian cancer is 60%. Thus, within the family, some women with the mutant gene will have only breast cancer, some only ovarian cancer, some will have both and some will have neither. Males with the mutant gene usually do not develop cancer but will, on average, transmit the mutant gene to 50% of their offspring. Thus, a female related to other affected females through unaffected males is still at high risk.

In Figure 2.25, the consultand is concerned about her family history of cancer. Multiple women have had variable combinations of breast and/or ovarian cancer and this pattern would be highly suspicious of familial breast/ovarian cancer. DNA analysis of the *BRCA1* gene in an affected woman will confirm that this is the case. The woman can then be offered presymptomatic genetic testing and, if this is found to be positive, she can be offered appropriate screening. Counselling of other family members at risk will be required and the family should be referred to the regional genetics centre.[1]

Reference

1.   British Society for Human Genetics. Directory of UK Genetics Centres [www.bshg.org.uk/Directory/UKdirectory.htm].

Section 3

Clinical case scenarios

Clinical case scenarios

Introduction

This section applies the knowledge gained in the previous two sections to clinical situations.

Case 1: Unexpected finding at amniocentesis

SITUATION

An expectant mother underwent amniocentesis because of an elevated screening risk for Down syndrome and the cytogenetic laboratory has noted an unusual appearance of a chromosome (Figure 3.1). Which chromosome is causing concern? What is the significance of this finding?

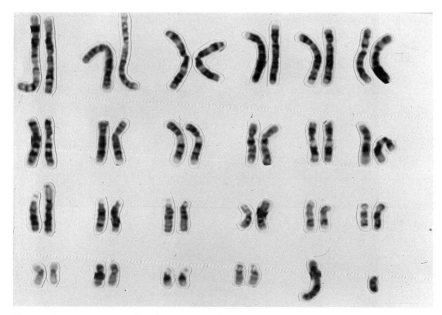

Figure 3.1 Karyotype for interpretation

CLINICAL RESPONSE

The short arm of chromosome 13 is longer than normal. The short arms of chromosomes 13–15, 21 and 22 are quite variable in length and reflect the number of copies of duplicated ribosomal genes in these areas. This is thus suspected to be a chromosomal variant or polymorphism of no clinical significance. This can be confirmed by checking the parents' blood karyotypes and finding that a healthy parent has the same chromosomal variant.

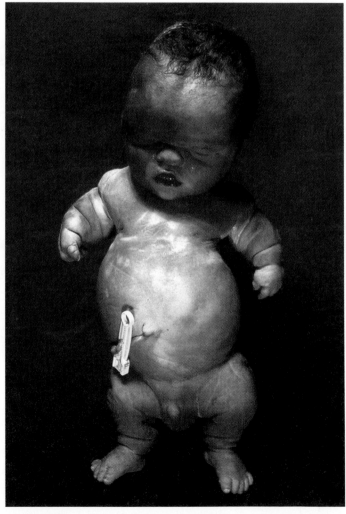

Figure 3.2 Lethal short-limbed skeletal dysplasia

Case 2: Lethal short-limbed skeletal dysplasia

SITUATION

Polyhydramnios in an otherwise uneventful pregnancy led to detailed ultrasound scanning. This revealed marked shortening of the limbs and the child was stillborn (Figure 3.2). What must the clinician do in this situation?

CLINICAL RESPONSE

There are multiple causes of lethal skeletal dysplasia. Some have high recurrence risks and some have low recurrence risks. A full body X-ray is crucial for distinguishing these different types and a DNA sample can also be extremely useful in confirming the suspected diagnosis. DNA can be extracted at postmortem from cardiac blood, a sample of liver or spleen or from cultured skin fibroblasts. Skin fibroblasts can still be grown from a skin biopsy as late as 3–4 days after death. Ideally, a full postmortem examination should be performed but, if the parents refuse consent, they will often allow an X-ray and a cardiac blood sample. For couples with a high risk of recurrence, prenatal reassurance can be offered by means of serial detailed ultrasound scans to monitor long-bone growth.

Case 3: Family history of Down syndrome

SITUATION

In the obstetric clinic a primigravida at 10 weeks of gestation reports that her cousin in America has just had a baby with Down syndrome. What action is required?

CLINICAL RESPONSE

Clinically, it is impossible to distinguish the more common low-risk trisomy 21 from the less common potentially high-risk translocation Down syndrome. Full details of the affected child (name, date of birth, mother's name and address) should be taken and the regional genetics centre will contact the American centre to see if chromosomal analysis has been performed. If it has and the result is trisomy 21 our patient can be reassured that she has only the general population risk and offered standard first- or second-trimester Down syndrome screening. If the affected child has translocation Down syndrome then our patient needs an urgent blood chromosome analysis to ensure that she is not a translocation carrier. If she were, the couple would need to be counselled and offered prenatal diagnosis. If contact with the American centre is not possible then, despite the low risk, blood chromosome analysis should be performed on our patient to exclude a translocation.

Case 4: Family history of Huntington's disease

SITUATION

An elderly primigravida (38 years of age) is concerned about her family history of Huntington's disease, which affects her father and affected her paternal grandmother (now deceased) (Figure 3.3). Using the web-based resource Online Mendelian Inheritance in Man (Appendix 1), is it possible to determine the mode of inheritance of Huntington's disease? What is her risk at 38 years of age? What is the risk to the fetus? Are DNA based tests available to help clarify these risks?

CLINICAL RESPONSE

Huntington's disease is inherited as an autosomal dominant trait with age-dependent expression. The gene is located near the tip of the short arm of chromosome 4 and each affected person thus has one mutant gene and a normal gene on the opposite copy of chromosome 4. The risk to our patient that she has inherited the mutant gene from her father is one in two. The condition may present in childhood but this is unusual and onset

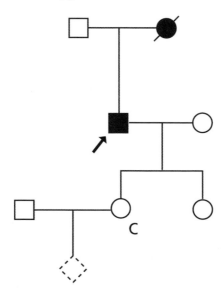

Figure 3.3 Family history of Huntington's disease

in the 40s or 50s is more usual. Thus, even though our patient is currently healthy, she is too young to significantly reduce her risk from one in two. The risk to her fetus is one-half of her own risk or one in four.

A DNA test for Huntington's disease is available and affected patients show a length mutation with the mutant gene being larger in size than the normal gene. This length mutation is unstable and may change in size on transmission, especially from a male. The couple needs careful counselling to ensure that they understand the implications of DNA testing and this will usually be undertaken by the regional genetics centre. If she does not carry the mutant gene for Huntington's disease then the risk to the fetus is negligible and prenatal testing for this condition is not indicated.

Case 5: Family history of Duchenne muscular dystrophy

SITUATION

In his referral letter to the obstetric booking clinic, the general practitioner notes that the pregnant woman's brother died of Duchenne muscular dystrophy and so he has measured her level of serum creatine kinase and found it to be within normal limits. Can she be reassured?

CLINICAL RESPONSE

This woman's pregnancy is at high risk of Duchenne muscular dystrophy, despite her normal level of serum creatine kinase, and she needs an urgent referral to the regional genetics centre to clarify the magnitude of this risk. Duchenne muscular dystrophy is inherited as an X-linked recessive trait and, in the absence of any other family history, the mother of an affected son has a two-thirds risk of being a carrier. If her levels of serum creatine kinase are elevated, this will confirm that she is a carrier, although normal levels are found in one-third of known carriers. Without creatine kinase data, her daughter will have a one in three chance of being a carrier and thus will have a one in six chance that a male pregnancy will be affected. As for her mother, an elevated level of creatine kinase will raise her risk of being a carrier but a normal level will not exclude the chance that she is a carrier. This is further confounded by measuring levels of creatine kinase during pregnancy, when the levels are reduced in both carriers and noncarriers.

In the genetics clinic, information from the family tree and creatine kinase levels will be combined to give a risk to the pregnancy and this will be supplemented by DNA analysis, which will be helpful for both precise carrier detection and prenatal diagnosis.

Case 6: Unexplained high level of maternal serum alphafetoprotein

SITUATION

Routine antenatal MSα-FP screening reveals a high level but detailed ultrasound scans are normal.

Clinical response

MSα-FP can be elevated for a variety of causes. One of the most common causes is an underestimated gestation. The ultrasound scans will exclude anencephaly, encephalocele and the majority of cases of spina bifida. They will also exclude a delayed miscarriage, anterior abdominal wall defects and teratoma. Rarer identifiable causes include fetal skin defects, placental haemangioma, congenital nephrotic syndrome and maternal hereditary persistence of α-FP.

Unexplained elevations of MSα-FP are associated with an increased risk of spontaneous miscarriage, stillbirth, low birth weight and perinatal death and thus these pregnancies merit follow-up.

Case 7: Family history of siblings with Goldenhar syndrome

SITUATION

A colleague asks your advice about an Australian family with Goldenhar syndrome. This affects a brother and sister and their aunt is expecting her first child.

CLINICAL RESPONSE

Online Mendelian Inheritance in Man (Appendix 1) can be used to look at the genetics and clinical features of Goldenhar syndrome. This reveals that Goldenhar syndrome is usually not inherited and hence two affected persons in the same family would be most unusual. This would bring the diagnosis into question and urgent assessment by a clinical geneticist is required. (In this family, the children had learning disabilities and dysmorphic features caused by an inherited translocation.)

This family emphasises the need to be really secure about the diagnosis before proceeding with genetic counselling and prenatal diagnosis. Assessment of clinical syndromes can be especially difficult as only rarely does an affected person have every clinical feature. Terms such as atypical case or *forme fruste* are commonly associated with an incorrect diagnosis.

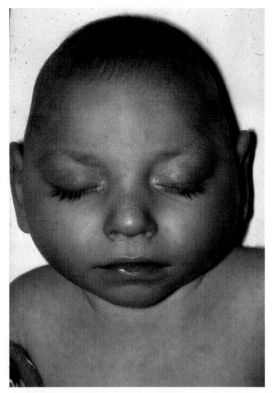

Figure 3.4 Microcephaly

Case 8: Family history of microcephaly

SITUATION

The pedigree of a family with a child (Figure 3.4) with microcephaly is shown in Figure 3.5.

CLINICAL RESPONSE

Microcephaly reflects defective brain growth and has multiple causes. In this family the parents are blood relatives (first cousins) and this makes the diagnosis of autosomal recessive microcephaly highly likely. DNA testing to confirm this is not yet available. The couple would be counselled that this is the likeliest diagnosis and that in this event the recurrence risk is one in four. Prenatal diagnosis by serial ultrasound measurements of

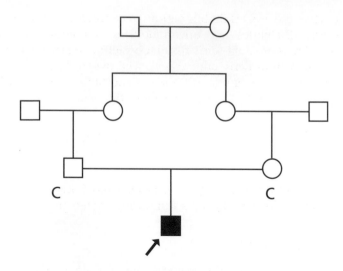

Figure 3.5 Family history of microcephaly (affected child is shown in Figure 3.4)

fetal head growth could be offered in a future pregnancy but the reduced head growth may not be evident until late in the pregnancy.

Other causes of microcephaly include congenital infection (rubella, cytomegalovirus or toxoplasmosis), birth trauma, chromosomal imbalance, fetal alcohol syndrome and maternal phenylketonuria. The latter needs to be considered in families with affected siblings with microcephaly before concluding that autosomal recessive microcephaly is the cause.

Case 9: Unexpected finding at amniocentesis

SITUATION

Amniocentesis was performed in view of an elevated maternal serum screening risk of Down syndrome and the karyotype revealed 47,XXY.

CLINICAL RESPONSE

This is the karyotype of Klinefelter syndrome (see Figure 2.1). The parents will need careful counselling in order to make an informed decision about the pregnancy. The older medical textbooks gave an ill-informed picture and information from unselected newborn surveys reveals that most children with Klinefelter syndrome are clinically normal. There is a 10–20 point reduction in verbal skills but performance scores are usually normal and learning disabilities are uncommon. As an adult infertility is invariable unless there is mosaicism and testosterone replacement therapy will be required from early adolescence. The overall birth incidence of Klinefelter syndrome is one in 1000 males and the recurrence risk for a family does not appear to be increased above this general population risk.

Case 10: Family history of Down syndrome

SITUATION

At booking, a mother reports that her brother has Down syndrome and she was told that she would need a test during any pregnancy.

CLINICAL RESPONSE

The key is to determine whether this is the more common trisomy 21 type of Down syndrome or the less common chromosomal translocation form. If her brother has trisomy 21, her recurrence risk is not increased above the general population risk (see Table 2.1), whereas if he has a translocation her pregnancy may be at substantial risk.

The local regional genetics centre should be contacted with the full name, date of birth and address in early childhood for the affected brother. Their records will show if he has trisomy 21 or a translocation. If he has a translocation, family members might already have been tested. This was the case with this family and the sister was known to carry a translocation involving chromosome 21. In this situation there is a high risk (15%) of Down syndrome for her pregnancy and prenatal diagnosis by amniocentesis or chorionic villus sampling should be offered. In this situation, a screening test using maternal blood is completely inappropriate.

Case 11: Importance of genetic ancestry

SITUATION

At booking, a healthy Cypriot mother is found to have a hypochromic microcytic anaemia.

CLINICAL RESPONSE

Most commonly, a hypochromic microcytic anaemia in pregnancy will be due to iron deficiency. Occasionally, there are other causes and this might be suspected in this situation given the genetic ancestry of the mother.

One in six Cypriots are carriers for beta-thalassaemia. These carriers are healthy but have microcytosis (with a mean corpuscular volume less than 80 fl) and a low mean cell haemoglobin (mean corpuscular haemoglobin less than 27 pg/cell). In contrast to iron deficiency anaemia, the iron stores are normal and haemoglobin A_2 is increased (greater than 3.5%).

If carrier status for beta-thalassaemia is confirmed, the woman's partner will also need to be tested. If both are carriers then the pregnancy has a one in four risk of beta-thalassaemia, which causes a severe chronic anaemia with a need for recurrent blood transfusions. Over 120 different mutations in the beta-globin gene cluster may be responsible but, in each population group, a subset of mutations is particularly common. DNA analysis can be used for prenatal diagnosis once the causative mutations in a family are known. Other family members also need to be offered genetic counselling and carrier testing.

Beta-thalassaemia carriers are particularly frequent in Mediterranean countries and South-East Asia. Other examples of conditions where the genetic ancestry is important are sickle cell disease, alpha-thalassaemia and Tay-Sachs disease.

Sickle cell disease is inherited as an autosomal recessive trait and is caused by a specific mutation in the beta-globin gene. It is especially prevalent in people of African or Caribbean descent, people from the Mediterranean, India and the Middle East. Routine haematological tests are normal in carriers and the haematology laboratory will perform specific tests if alerted by the clinician. If both parents are carriers there is a one in four risk that the fetus will have sickle cell disease. This is a severe chronic haemolytic anaemia with associated infarctions due to vascular obstruction. Prenatal diagnosis can be offered by DNA analysis.

Alpha-thalassaemia is inherited as an autosomal recessive trait and is caused by a variety of mutations in the alpha-globin gene cluster. The severe form of alpha-thalassaemia is caused by a complete lack of alpha-globin genes. In this case there is a profound *in utero* anaemia with hydrops fetalis and intrauterine or early neonatal death. The carrier parents of this severe form show a hypochromic microcytic anaemia, which needs to be distinguished from iron deficiency anaemia and beta-thalassaemia carrier status. Carriers of the severe form of alpha-thalassaemia are particularly frequent in South-East Asia. Prenatal diagnosis for at-risk pregnancies can be offered by DNA analysis.

Tay-Sachs disease needs to be considered when the parents are Ashkenazi Jews. This is inherited as an autosomal recessive trait and results in a progressive incurable neurodegeneration in childhood. Carrier parents are healthy but have reduced serum and leucocyte beta-*N*-acetylhexosaminidase A levels. Prenatal diagnosis can be offered by enzyme analysis or DNA analysis.

Case 12: Never say never

SITUATION

At a prepregnancy clinic, a prospective mother raises her concerns about a limb defect in her nephew (Figure 3.6).

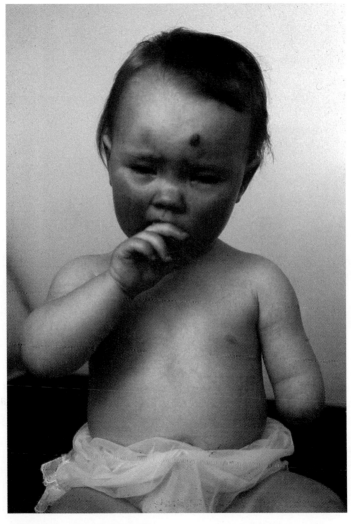

Figure 3.6 Transverse limb defect

CLINICAL RESPONSE

The limb defect in this child is a typical transverse amputation defect. Most, if not all, are believed to be due to *in utero* amputations by strands of amnion produced by premature rupture of the amnion. If the chorion is also involved, there may be a history of leakage of liquor and the child may also show congenital deformations due to oligohydramnios. The amniotic bands may produce a variety of other defects, including asymmetric facial clefts.

The general population frequency is one in 5000 and in this situation the prospective mother would be reassured that her risk was low but not nonexistent (as we all have the general population risk). Further reassurance can be offered if required in a future pregnancy by detailed ultrasound scanning.

Case 13: Unexpected finding at amniocentesis

SITUATION

At amniocentesis, in view of an increased maternal serum screening risk for Down syndrome, an apparently balanced chromosomal translocation between chromosomes 11 and 22 is detected (Figure 3.7). What action is indicated?

CLINICAL RESPONSE

The cytogenetic report included the word 'apparently' as the lower limit of resolution of DNA loss or gain with the light microscope is 4 Mb. In the creation of a translocation, chromosomal breaks occur and DNA may be damaged or lost at the breakpoints. In order to exclude this possibility the first step is to check the parental chromosomes. If a healthy parent carries the same translocation then the couple can be reassured that the fetus will not be affected by the chromosomal change. The couple will need counselling with regard to the possibility of chromosomally unbalanced offspring in future pregnancies and options for prenatal diagnosis. Other family members who might also be carriers of the translocation will need to be offered tests. If neither parent has the translocation then there is a small risk that the fetus may have an abnormal phenotype. Detailed ultrasound scanning is indicated to exclude congenital malformations. If malformations are present this would make a chromosomal imbalance highly likely and termination of pregnancy would need to be considered.

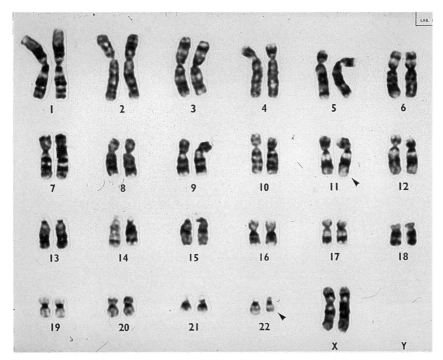

Figure 3.7 Karyotype of an apparently balanced translocation between chromosomes 11 and 22 (arrowed)

Case 14: Inherited limb abnormality

SITUATION

At booking, the midwife notes a limb abnormality in the mother (Figure 3.8) and some of her relatives (Figure 3.9). What is the diagnosis in the mother? What is the mode of inheritance?

CLINICAL RESPONSE

The mother shows soft tissue syndactyly and the family tree is typical of autosomal dominant inheritance. The mother and other relatives are otherwise healthy but the extent of the syndactyly varies from one family member to another. In counselling this family, the range and features shown by family members is helpful. Autosomal dominant traits often show variation in the degree of involvement between different family members (variable expression). The website Online Mendelian Inheritance

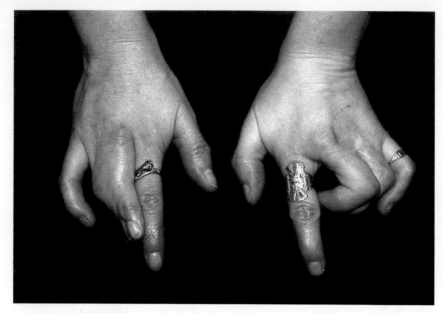

Figure 3.8 Syndactyly

in Man lists multiple forms of syndactyly inherited in this fashion but as yet few of the genes have been identified and thus DNA testing is not useful for genetic counselling.

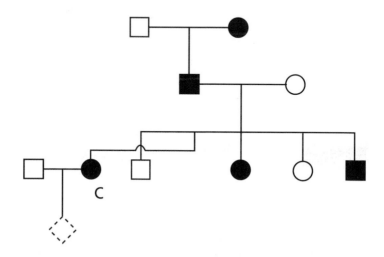

Figure 3.9 Family history of syndactyly (consultand is shown in Figure 3.8)

Case 15: Multiple congenital abnormalities

SITUATION

At routine ultrasound scanning, multiple congenital malformations are detected and the parents opted for termination of pregnancy (Figure 3.10). What features are evident? Is a syndrome diagnosis possible?

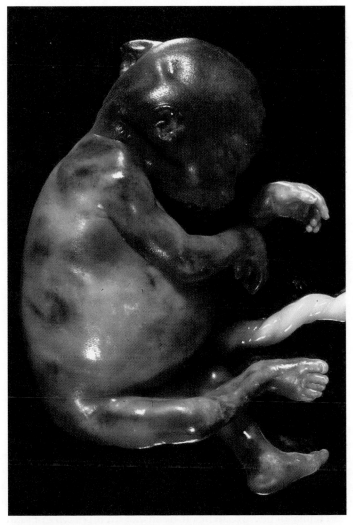

Figure 3.10 Fetus with multiple congenital abnormalities

CLINICAL RESPONSE

The fetus has an encephalocele, polydactyly (on the little finger/toe side – called postaxial) and a swollen abdomen, which, at postmortem, was shown to be caused by polycystic kidneys.

Using the facilities of the Dysmorphic Human–Mouse Homology Database (Appendix 1), a syndromic diagnosis can be identified.

Under 'feature selection', the three main clinical features are noted. Posterior encephalocele, meningocele is under the subheading of 'brain, general abnormalities', which is under the heading of 'cranium'. Postaxial polydactyly is under the subheading of 'fingers, general abnormalities', which is under the heading of 'hands/forefeet'. Multiple renal cysts is listed under the subheading of 'kidneys, general abnormalities', which is under the heading of 'urinary system'. A search on the combination of these three features reveals two potential matches and of these Meckel–Gruber syndrome is the most likely. By clicking on this syndrome name, further features are highlighted and these can be looked for in the postmortem report to confirm the clinical diagnosis.

Using the website, Online Mendelian Inheritance in Man, the genetic information can be determined for this syndrome. This shows that the condition is inherited as an autosomal recessive trait and that several genes have been identified which can cause the condition. Analysis of these genes is not yet routinely available and thus the parents need to be counselled that the recurrence risk is one in four and prenatal diagnosis can be offered by detailed ultrasound scanning to look for the clinical features. Experience in prenatal diagnosis for this condition can be reviewed by searching the PubMed database (Appendix 1) using the key words 'Meckel–Gruber syndrome' and 'prenatal diagnosis'.

Case 16: Family history of cystic fibrosis

SITUATION

At booking, a mother's partner is noted to have a child by a previous relationship who has cystic fibrosis (Figure 3.11). What action is necessary?

CLINICAL RESPONSE

Cystic fibrosis is inherited as an autosomal recessive disorder and thus both parents of the affected child must be carriers. The mother in the antenatal clinic has no family history of cystic fibrosis and thus she has the general population risk of one in 22. The combined risk to her pregnancy is thus her chance of being a carrier (one in 22) multiplied by her partner's risk of being a carrier (one in one – must be a carrier) multiplied by the

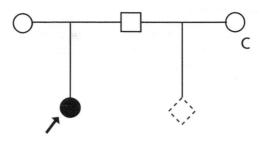

Figure 3.11 Family history of cystic fibrosis

chance that two carriers will both hand on the underactive gene (one in four). The combined risk to the pregnancy is thus one in 88. This risk can be modified by DNA testing of the pregnant mother. The commonly used mutation screen for cystic fibrosis detects 90% of mutations. If the mother has a negative screen her residual chance of being a carrier will fall to one in 220 (one in 22 multiplied by one in ten or 10%) and the risk to her pregnancy will fall to one in 880 (one in 220 × 1 × one in four). If she is shown on DNA testing to be a carrier then the risk to her pregnancy rises to one in four and the couple can be offered prenatal diagnosis by DNA analysis.

Case 17: Previous obstetric history of trisomy 13

SITUATION

After an uneventful pregnancy, a 25-year-old mother was delivered of an infant with trisomy 13 (Figure 3.12). What counselling should be provided?

CLINICAL RESPONSE

Trisomy 13 (Patau syndrome) occurs once in every 5000 live births and is the least common autosomal trisomy. As with other autosomal trisomies, the risk increases with maternal age but, in common with them, most affected pregnancies occur in younger mothers as they account for the majority of pregnancies. Either the egg or the sperm will have had two copies of chromosome 13, thus resulting in 47 chromosomes in total with trisomy of 13. Occasionally, a translocation involving chromosome 13 is found and thus all patients need cytogenetic confirmation even if the clinical diagnosis is secure. Provided that a

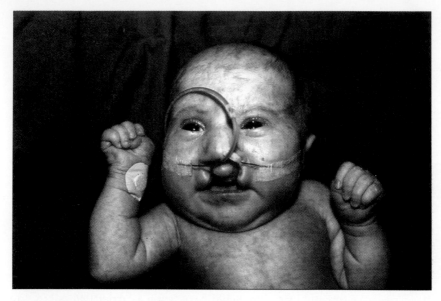

Figure 3.12 Patau syndrome – trisomy 13

translocation is not involved the recurrence risk is less than 1% and reassurance can be provided by chromosome analysis following amniocentesis or chorionic villus sampling in a future pregnancy.

Multiple malformations are usual in trisomy 13. As seen in this child, these include closely spaced eyes (hypotelorism) reflecting an under-lying brain malformation (holoprosencephaly), small eyes (micro-phthalmia) and bilateral cleft lip and palate. Congenital heart disease is usual and 50% of affected infants die within 1 month. Only 10% survive beyond the first year and these children show profound developmental delay.

Case 18: Previous obstetric history of hydrocephalus

SITUATION

A couples' first son has hydrocephalus (Figure 3.13) and they have learned that there is a distant family history of the same condition (Figure 3.14). What type of inheritance does the pedigree suggest? Is there a known single gene form of hydrocephalus inherited in this fashion?

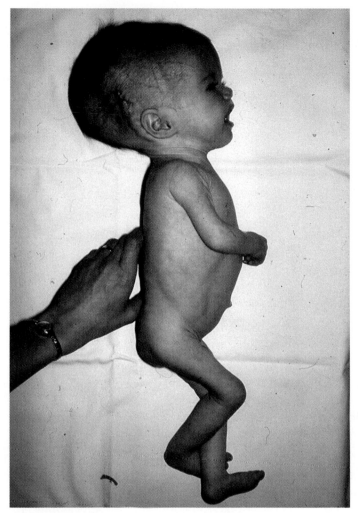

Figure 3.13 Hydrocephalus

CLINICAL RESPONSE

Hydrocephalus may be secondary to a neural tube defect or isolated, as in this child. Identifiable causes of isolated hydrocephalus include intra-cranial haemorrhage, fetal infection and multifactorial, X-linked recessive or autosomal recessive inheritance.

The family tree shows only affected males who are linked by unaffected females. This is characteristic of X-linked recessive inheritance. This would

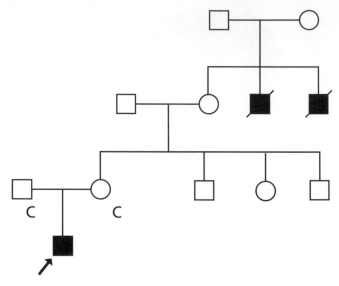

Figure 3.14 Family history of hydrocephalus (proband is shown in Figure 3.13)

make the diagnosis of X-linked recessive hydrocephalus highly likely. Using the website Online Mendelian Inheritance in Man", the genetic information can be determined for this condition by searching on 'hydrocephalus, X-linked recessive'. The top condition in this search is hydrocephalus due to stenosis of the aqueduct of Sylvius and by clicking on this more information can be gleaned. This entry has the number #307000. The # sign means that a gene has been identified for the condition and the number is a unique identifier for each condition. Numbers starting with 3 are for X-linked conditions (those beginning with 2 are for autosomal recessive conditions and those beginning with 1 are for autosomal dominant conditions).

Clinical features that support this diagnosis are characteristic hypoplastic flexed thumbs in a male with postmortem evidence of stenosis of the aqueduct of Sylvius and absence of the pyramids from sections of the medulla. The condition is caused by mutations in the L1 cell adhesion molecule gene (*L1CAM*), which is located near to the tip of the long arm of the X chromosome (in band Xq28). DNA analysis can be used to confirm the clinical diagnosis and to identify carrier females within the family.

The mother of the affected child in Figure 3.14 must be a carrier as she has other affected relatives. The alternative explanation of multiple new mutations is highly unlikely and 50% of her sons are expected to be affected. Prenatal diagnosis can be offered by DNA analysis. Prenatal diagnosis by serial ultrasound scanning may be possible but might not be diagnostic until very late in pregnancy.

Case 19: Maternal congenital heart disease

SITUATION

A mother in her first pregnancy reports that she had a 'hole in the heart' repaired when she was a baby. What is the clinical significance?

CLINICAL RESPONSE

Overall congenital heart disease affects eight in every 1000 births and many different causes can be identified. Most (85%) are inherited as multifactorial conditions and this diagnosis is reached by excluding other diagnoses including congenital infection (2%), chromosomal disorders (10%, including microdeletions, especially of 22q11) and single-gene disorders (3%).

The term 'hole in the heart' is used indiscriminately and this woman's medical records are required to determine the type of congenital heart disease and the nature of the operative correction. There will be implications for her own medical management during the pregnancy and genetic implications for her fetus. The genetic risk will depend upon the cause of the condition. For multifactorial congenital heart disease the overall risk to the fetus is one in 25 (4%) and detailed ultrasound scanning at 18–20 weeks of gestation could be offered. A recurrence of congenital heart disease in this situation would not necessarily be of the same type or same severity as that of the mother.

Case 20: Family history of problems

SITUATION

At birth a child is noted to be hypotonic and is transferred to the special care baby unit (Figure 3.15). A family history is taken (Figure 3.16). What is the likely diagnosis? What is the recurrence risk?

CLINICAL RESPONSE

Neonatal hypotonia and a family history of individuals with cataracts and muscle weakness is suggestive of myotonic dystrophy. The mother of the child needs to be carefully examined, as it is easy to overlook mild

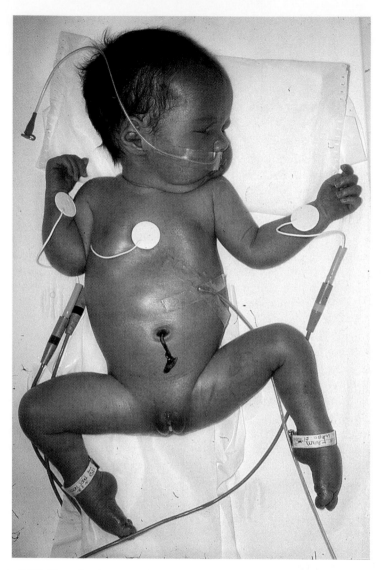

Figure 3.15 Hypotonic neonate

symptoms (expressionless face, myotonia or delayed muscle relaxation, for example after shaking hands). DNA testing of an affected individual will confirm the diagnosis by showing a mutant *DMPK* gene that is larger than normal (see Figure 1.23).

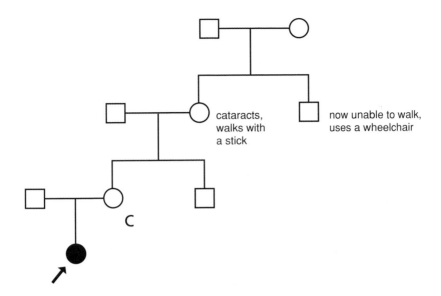

Figure 3.16 Family history of hypotonic neonate shown in Figure 3.15

cataracts,
walks with
a stick

now unable to walk,
uses a wheelchair

C

Affected neonates have invariably received the mutant gene from their mothers and the gene will have been markedly increased in size at transmission. The condition is inherited as an autosomal dominant trait and thus the mother has a one in two chance of handing on the normal gene and a one in two chance of handing on the mutant gene. Of the children who receive the mutant gene in this situation, 50% will be affected in later life and 50% will present as newborns with hypotonia and subsequent learning disabilities or neonatal death. Prenatal diagnosis by DNA analysis can be offered. The children with newborn presentations always show large gene length mutations but there is not an exact correlation with timing and severity of clinical symptoms and careful genetic counselling is required.

Case 21: Unexpected finding at amniocentesis

SITUATION

An amniocentesis is performed, as a mother has an increased screening risk of Down syndrome. The result is reported as 46,XY/46,XX.

CLINICAL RESPONSE

The result would indicate two cell lines or mosaicism and this would need to be discussed with the cytogenetic laboratory who will be able to provide information on the relative proportions of each cell line and the likely clinical significance. In true mosaicism (that is, mosaicism in the fetus or placenta) the abnormal cell line is usually present in several different cultures set up from the original sample, whereas in pseudomosaicism (that is, an *in vitro* artefact) only one culture is involved.

Single cell pseudomosaicism is found in about 3% of amniocenteses and as there is a less than 1% chance that this represents true mosaicism no further action is generally taken. Pseudomosaicism in multiple cells is found in about 1% of all amniocenteses. Repeat amniocentesis or fetal blood sampling may be required, especially if few cells were available for analysis and if the abnormality is seen in liveborn infants.

True mosaicism is found in 0.25% of all amniocenteses and in about 25% of these the phenotype is abnormal. Fetal blood sampling and detailed ultrasound scanning for malformations may be required.

46,XY/46,XX mosaicism almost invariably represents maternal cell contamination with a normal male fetus. The chance of maternal cell contamination is greatly reduced if a stilette is used in the needle and if the first few drops of amniotic fluid withdrawn are discarded.

Case 22: Previous obstetric history of a fetus with multiple congenital malformations

SITUATION

A healthy non-consanguineous couple with no family history were in mid-pregnancy when an elevated level of MSα-FP led to a detailed ultrasound scan. Multiple congenital malformations were apparent and the couple elected for termination of pregnancy. At postmortem, the fetus had an anterior abdominal wall defect (exomphalos), congenital heart disease and a missing left kidney (Figure 3.17).

CLINICAL RESPONSE

Congenital malformations may be caused by a variety of factors. Skin fibroblasts grown from fascia lata from the fetus gave a normal result and the clinical geneticist was unable to identify a specific syndrome. In this situation, the specific risk of recurrence is 2–5% in addition to the general population risk for a congenital malformation of 2–3%. Reassurance by means of detailed ultrasound scanning might be offered during subsequent pregnancies.

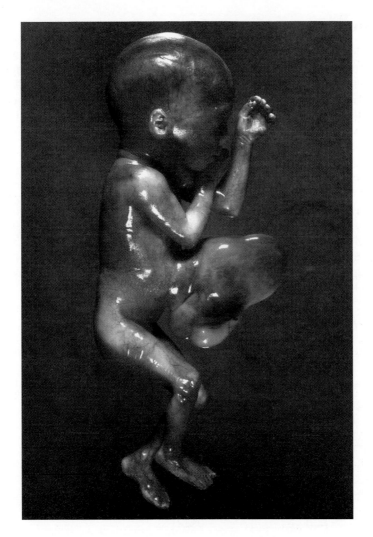

Figure 3.17 Fetus with multiple congenital abnormalities

Case 23: Accidental X-ray in early pregnancy

SITUATION

A general practitioner asks for advice as one of his patients had a chest X-ray while on holiday abroad and now realises that she was three weeks pregnant when the X-ray was performed. What advice should be given to the general practitioner and his patient?

An accidental diagnostic X-ray (of 0.01 Gy or less) during early pregnancy results in a total added risk of one in 1000 to the fetus for congenital malformation, learning disabilities or childhood cancer. Neither termination of pregnancy nor amniocentesis is indicated. The fetal risk increases in relation to the dose of X-rays. Termination is generally advised if a fetus less than 8 weeks is exposed to more than 0.25 Gy (25 rads). Exposure to 2–4 Gy usually results in female sterility.

Case 24: Genetic mimicry

SITUATION

At booking, a mother reports that her husband has poor vision due to retinitis pigmentosa. There is no other family history of the condition (Figure 3.18). What is the inheritance of retinitis pigmentosa? What is the risk to her pregnancy?

CLINICAL RESPONSE

The Online Mendelian Inheritance in Man website reveals multiple entries for retinitis pigmentosa. Some (15%) are inherited as autosomal dominant traits, some (70%) as autosomal recessive traits and some

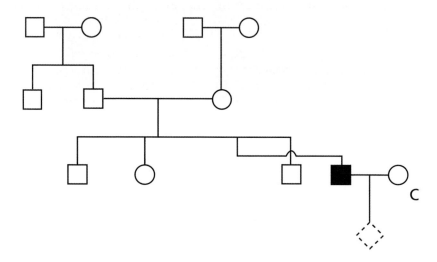

Figure 3.18 Family history of retinitis pigmentosa

(15%) as X-linked recessive traits. This situation where clinically similar conditions may be caused by mutations in a variety of genes is termed genetic heterogeneity or genetic mimicry. In this family, there is no family history to suggest any mode of inheritance. The husband could have a new mutation for an autosomal dominant condition, he could be an affected autosomal recessive homozygote or he could be affected with an X-linked recessive form. In view of the multiple genes involved, it is not yet practicable to determine which gene is involved in every case and empiric figures are used for counselling. The risk of retinitis pigmentosa for the pregnancy is one in eight. This reflects the combined risk, which is high if he has an autosomal dominant trait and much lower if he has an autosomal recessive or X-linked condition.

In the absence of a known molecular basis prenatal diagnosis is not possible.

Case 25: Previous obstetric history of an intrauterine death with cystic hygroma

SITUATION

A healthy non-consanguineous couple had a previous intrauterine death with a cystic hygroma. What is the risk of recurrence?

CLINICAL RESPONSE

About 50% of cystic hygromas are associated with Turner syndrome (45,X; see Figure 2.2) and this may also be seen with trisomies of 21, 18 and 13. Hence, chromosome analysis on the child was indicated. This may be possible on fibroblast culture from fascia lata even 3–4 days after death. If chromosome analysis failed or was not undertaken then it would be necessary to perform parental karyotypes to exclude a balanced chromosomal rearrangement. Unless the cause was an autosomal trisomy, the risk of recurrence is low and reassurance could be given by means of ultrasound scanning in a future pregnancy.

Appendix 1.
Sources of genetic information

Genetic conditions and syndromes are numerous and so medical geneticists rely heavily on databases of genetic information in addition to the standard medical literature. There are many web-based resources but some of the most useful are:

On-line Mendelian Inheritance in Man

www3.ncbi.nlm.nih.gov/entrez/query.fcgi?db=OMIM

Contains detailed genetic information on disorders caused by mutations in single genes and links to other relevant databases. Many of the reviews contain a clinical synopsis.

Dysmorphic Human–Mouse Homology Database

www.hgmp.mrc.ac.uk/DHMHD/dysmorph.html

Developed at the Clinical Genetics and Fetal Medicine Unit of the Institute of Child Health in London.

This site is useful for viewing features of a named syndrome or a particular chromosomal abnormality and can be used to help in diagnosing a syndrome by searching for the particular symptoms and signs that affect a patient with an unidentified condition.

PubMed

www.ncbi.nlm.nih.gov/entrez/query.fcgi?db=PubMed

Allows literature searches on key words and is thus particularly useful for finding recent publications in an area of interest.

Directory of UK Genetics Centres

www.bshg.org.uk/Directory/UKdirectory.htm

British Society for Human Genetics Directory of UK Genetics Centres. Contact details for local regional genetics service can be found at this website.

Further reading

Harper PS. *Practical Genetic Counselling*. 6th ed. Oxford: Oxford University Press; 2004.

Mueller R, Young I. *Emery's Elements of Genetics*. 11th ed. Edinburgh: Churchill Livingstone; 2001.

Rimoin DL, Connor JM, Pyeritz RE, Korf BR, editors. *Emery and Rimoin's Principles and Practice of Medical Genetics*. 4th ed. Edinburgh: Churchill Livingstone; 2002.

Index

adenine (A) 3
adults
  chromosome analysis 30
  DNA analysis 29
Alagille syndrome 11
alleles 10
alphafetoprotein, maternal serum
  (MSα-FP)
  Down syndrome 41, 42
  neural tube defects 46–7
  unexplained high level 74
alpha-globin gene mutations 78
alpha-thalassaemia 78
amniocentesis 39, 40
  case scenarios 69–70, 76–7, 80–1,
    91–2
  Down syndrome risk and 44
amniotic bands 80
anaemia, hypochromic microcytic
  77–8
anencephaly 48, 56
  maternal serum screening 47
Angelman syndrome 11
aniridia syndrome 11
antenatal screening risk *see* maternal
  screening risk
aqueduct (of Sylvius) stenosis 88
Ashkenazi Jews 78
atypical case 74
autosomal disorders 10, 11
autosomal dominant disorders 11
  inheritance 12, 13, 22, 23
  learning difficulties 62
autosomal recessive disorders 11
  inheritance 12–13, 15, 22, 23
  learning difficulties 62

autosomes 6

base pairs 3
beta-globin gene mutations 78
beta human chorionic
  gonadotrophin, free (FβhCG)
  41, 43, 44
beta-thalassaemia 78
BRCA1 gene mutations 65–6
breast cancer, familial 65–6
British Society for Human Genetics,
  Directory of UK Genetics
  Centres 98

cancer 18–19, 65–6
carriers 14
  alpha-thalassaemia 78
  balanced translocations 38–41
  beta-thalassaemia 78
  cystic fibrosis 51, 84–5
  Down syndrome translocation
    52–4
  Duchenne muscular dystrophy
    (DMD) 59–60, 73
  fragile X syndrome 62, 63
  myotonic dystrophy 61, 91
  obligate 24
  sickle cell disease 78
centromeres 4
CFTR gene mutations 51, 58
  antenatal screening 51
  DNA analysis 25, 26
  male infertility 35
children
  chromosome analysis 30
  DNA analysis 29

chorionic villus sampling (CVS)
    39–40
chromosomal disorders 6–10
    congenital malformations 64
    cystic hygroma 95
    learning difficulties 61–2
    numerical 6
    recurrent miscarriages 36–41
    somatic cell 18
    structural 6–10
    see also Down syndrome
chromosome analysis 28–9, 30
    unexpected findings 69–70, 76–7,
        80–1
chromosomes 3
cleft lip and palate 17, 86
codon 4
confidentiality 32
congenital heart disease, maternal
    89
congenital malformations 63–5
    aetiology 64
    multifactorial inheritance 17–18,
        64
    multiple 83–4, 92–3
consanguinity 22
consultand 30
counselling, genetic 31, 32
creatine (phospho)kinase (CPK),
    serum 59, 73
Cypriot descent 77–8
cystic fibrosis
    elevated maternal screening risk
        51
    family history 57–9, 84–5
    gene mutations see CFTR gene
        mutations
cystic hygroma 95
cytosine (C) 3

deletions, chromosomal 9–10, 11
delF508 (δF508) mutation 51, 58
    DNA analysis 23, 26
diabetes mellitus, maternal 64
diagnosis
    assessment of accuracy 74
    genetic disorders 30–1

diagnostic test, vs screening test 45
DiGeorge syndrome 11
Directory of UK Genetics Centres 98
dizygotic twins 16–17
DMPK gene 60–1, 90
DNA 3–4
    analysis 24–7, 29
    sampling methods 24, 71
dominant disorders 10, 11
Down syndrome (trisomy 21) 6, 7
    elevated maternal screening risk
        41–51
    family history 52–6, 71–2, 77
    first-trimester screening 43, 44
    learning difficulties 61–2
    maternal age-related risk 41
    second-trimester screening 41–4
    translocation 52–6, 71–2, 77
Duchenne muscular dystrophy
    (DMD) 59–60, 73
Dysmorphic Human–Mouse
    Homology Database 97
dystrophia myotonica see myotonic
    dystrophy

ectrodactyly 12
Edwards syndrome (trisomy 18) 6,
    7
encephalocele 56, 57
environmental factors 3, 15–16
epilepsy, maternal 64
ethnic origin, importance 77–8
extended family study 32, 40–1

family history 52–66
    congenital malformations 65
    cystic fibrosis 57–9, 84–5
    Down syndrome 52–6, 71–2, 77
    Duchenne muscular dystrophy
        59–60, 73
    Goldenhar syndrome 74
    Huntington's disease 72–3
    hydrocephalus 86–9
    learning difficulties 62–3
    microcephaly 75–6
    muscular dystrophy 59–61
    myotonic dystrophy 60–1, 89–91

neural tube defect 56–7
ovarian cancer 65–6
syndactyly 81–2
taking 20, 21
family tree (pedigree)
  drawing 19–20, 21
  interpretation 22–4
  number 32
fibroblasts, skin 71
FMR1 gene 62, 63
folic acid supplementation 56–7
forme fruste 74
fragile X syndrome 62–3

gene 4
genetic ancestry, importance 77–8
genetic assessment, referral for 30–2
genetic code 3–4
genetic counselling 31, 32
genetic disease
  common misconceptions 31
  diagnosis 30–1
  multifactorial 15–18
  somatic cell (cumulative) 18–19
  types 5–19
genetic mimicry (heterogeneity)
    94–5
Goldenhar syndrome 74
gonadal mosaicism 18
guanine (G) 3

heredity, common misconceptions 31
heterozygous 10
'hole in the heart,' maternal 89
holoprosencephaly 86
homozygous 10
horizontal pattern of inheritance 22,
    23
HPRT gene 13–14
  DNA analysis 27, 28
human chorionic gonadotrophin
    (hCG), maternal serum 41, 42
Huntington's disease 72–3
Hurler syndrome 12–13, 14
hydrocephalus 86–9
hypochromic microcytic anaemia
    77–8

hypotelorism 86
hypotonia, neonatal 61, 89–91

IDUA gene 12–13
infertility, genetic causes 35–6
inheritance 3–4
intrauterine death, previous, with
    cystic hygroma 95

karyotype 3
  analysis *see* chromosome analysis
  female 4
  male 5
kilobase (kb) 3
Klinefelter syndrome 35, 36, 76–7
knight's move pattern of inheritance
    22–4

L1 cell adhesion molecule 88
learning difficulties 61–3
Lesch–Nyhan syndrome 13–14, 16
  DNA analysis 27, 28
LICAM gene mutations 88
limb
  inherited abnormality 81–2
  transverse defect 79–80
locus 10

male infertility 35
maternal age, Down syndrome risk
    and 41
maternal illness, congenital
    malformations and 64
maternal screening risk, elevated
    41–51
  cystic fibrosis 51
  Down syndrome 41–6
  neural tube defect 46–51
Meckel–Gruber syndrome 84
megabase (Mb) 3
Mendelian disorders *see* single-gene
    disorders
microcephaly 75–6
microdeletion syndromes,
    chromosomal 10, 11
microphthalmia 86
Miller-Dieker lissencephaly 11

miscarriage
  chromosomal disorders 6
  procedure-related risk 40
  recurrent, genetic causes 36–41
monosomy X 6, 8
  see also Turner syndrome
monozygotic twins 16–17
mosaicism 18, 91–2
multifactorial disorders 15–18
  congenital malformations 17–18, 64
multiple congenital abnormalities 83–4, 92–3
multiples of the median (MOM), Down syndrome risk assessment 41, 42, 43
muscular dystrophy 59–61, 73
mutations 24–5
  length 24, 25
  point 24–5
  somatic cell 18
  unstable 25
myotonic dystrophy 60–1
  DNA analysis 25
  family history 89–91

nature *vs* nurture 3
neonates
  chromosome analysis 30
  DNA analysis 29
neural tube defect
  elevated maternal screening risk 46–51
  family history 56–7
  secular change in frequency 56
nuchal oedema, fetal 35, 37
nuchal translucency 44

oestriol, unconjugated 41
Online Mendelian Inheritance in Man 97
  case scenarios 72, 74, 81–2, 84, 88, 94–5
ovarian cancer, familial 65–6

Patau syndrome *see* trisomy 13
pedigree *see* family tree

phenylketonuria, maternal 64
polydactyly 20, 21, 22, 23
polymerase chain reaction (PCR) 25
Prader-Willi syndrome 11
pregnancy, accidental X-ray in early 93–4
pregnancy-associated plasma protein A (PAPP-A) 43, 44
premutations 62
prenatal diagnosis 27, 29, 30
  balanced translocations 39–40
  see also maternal screening risk, elevated
presymptomatic testing 27, 29
proband 30
pseudomosaicism 92
PubMed 84, 97

recessive disorders 10, 11
referral, for genetic assessment and counselling 30–2
regional genetics centres 30
retinitis pigmentosa 94–5
rhabdomyosarcoma 18
risk(s)
  communication to patients 45–6, 47–8
  independent 41, 52
  mutually exclusive 52
  thresholds, high and low 45, 46

screening test, *vs* diagnostic test 45
sex chromosomes 3, 6
  disorders 10, 11
short stature, Turner syndrome 36
sibship 22
sickle cell disease 78
single-gene disorders 10–15
  congenital malformations 64
  DNA analysis 24–7
  learning difficulties 62
skeletal dysplasia, short-limbed lethal 70, 71
skin fibroblasts 71
somatic cell genetic disorders 18–19
somatic mosaicism 18
spina bifida 56

closed 47, 50
 open 47, 48, 49
 prognosis 48–50
split-hand syndrome 12
syndactyly 81–2
syndromes 30–1
syndromic diagnosis 83–4

Tay-Sachs disease 78
telomeres 4
thalassaemias 78
thymine (T) 3
TP73L gene 12
trait 10
translocations 9, 10
 balanced 9, 38, 80–1
 Down syndrome 52–6, 71–2, 77
 in recurrent miscarriage 36–41
transverse limb defect 79–80
triploidy 6, 9
trisomy 13 (Patau syndrome) 6, 8
 previous obstetric history 85–6
trisomy 16 6
trisomy 18 6, 7
trisomy 21 *see* Down syndrome

tuberous sclerosis 62
Turner syndrome 6, 8
 cystic hygroma 95
 diagnosis in fetus/newborn 35–6,
  37, 38
 infertility 35–6
twins 16–17

variable expression 81–2

Williams syndrome 11
Wilms tumour 11

X chromosome 3, 4
X-linked disorders 11
X-linked dominant disorders 11
X-linked recessive disorders 11
 hydrocephalus 87–8
 inheritance 13–14, 17, 22–4
 learning difficulties 62
X-ray, in early pregnancy, accidental
  93–4

Y chromosome 3, 5
Y-linked inheritance 11